Care Work and Medical Travel

Anthropology of Well-Being
Individual, Community, Society

Series Editor: Ben G. Blount, PhD (SocioEcological Informatics)

Mission Statement
Well-being is central and important in people's daily lives and life history. This book series brings about understanding of what the complex concepts of well-being include. The concepts of quality of life, life satisfaction, and happiness will be explored and viewed at the individual level, the community level, and the level of society. The series encourages and promotes research into the concept of well-being, how it appears to be defined culturally, and how it is utilized across levels and across different social, economic, and ethnic groups. Understandings of how well-being promotes stability and resilience will also be critical to advances in understanding, as well as how well-being can be implemented as a goal in resisting vulnerabilities and in adaptation. Series books include monographs and edited collections by a range of academics, from rising scholars to experts in relevant fields.

Advisory Board Members
Steven Jacob, Kathleen Galvin, Carlos Garcia-Quijano, Cynthia Isenhour, and Richard Pollnac

Recent Titles in the Series
Care Work and Medical Travel: Exploring the Emotional Dimensions of Caring on the Move, by Cecilia Vindrola-Padros
Being Ethical among Vezo People: Fisheries, Livelihoods, and Conservation in Madagascar, by Frank Muttenzer
Tourism and Maternal Health: Customs, Beliefs, and Everyday Practices, by Allison Cantor
Competing Orders of Medical Care in Ethiopia: From Traditional Healers to Pharmaceutical Companies, by Pino Schirippa, translated by Ciaran Durkan
Well-Being as a Multidimensional Concept: Understanding Connections among Culture, Community, and Health, edited by Janet M. Page-Reeves

Care Work and Medical Travel

Exploring the Emotional Dimensions of Caring on the Move

Edited by
Cecilia Vindrola-Padros

LEXINGTON BOOKS
Lanham • Boulder • New York • London

Published by Lexington Books
An imprint of The Rowman & Littlefield Publishing Group, Inc.
4501 Forbes Boulevard, Suite 200, Lanham, Maryland 20706
www.rowman.com

6 Tinworth Street, London SE11 5AL, United Kingdom

Copyright © 2021 The Rowman & Littlefield Publishing Group, Inc.

All rights reserved. No part of this book may be reproduced in any form or by any electronic or mechanical means, including information storage and retrieval systems, without written permission from the publisher, except by a reviewer who may quote passages in a review.

British Library Cataloguing in Publication Information Available

Library of Congress Cataloging-in-Publication Data on File

Library of Congress Control Number: 2021932368

ISBN 978-1-7936-1886-3 (cloth)
ISBN 978-1-7936-1887-0 (electronic)

Contents

Exploring the Emotional Dimensions of Caring on the Move:
An Introduction ... 1
Cecilia Vindrola-Padros

1 Healing in the Diaspora: Hmong American and Hmong Lao
   Practices of Care ... 11
   Mai See Thao and Audrey Bochaton

2 Informal Caregiving in a Transnational Context: The Case of
   Canadian International Retirement Migrants in the United States ... 35
   Valorie A. Crooks and John Pickering

3 Care, Choice, and Cure: Exploring the Logics of Mobility of
   Patients with Breast Cancer in Italy and France ... 51
   Cinzia Greco

4 Providing High Quality Care: What Cross-border Medical
   Travel Can Teach Us ... 69
   Matthew Dalstrom

5 "Caring for" and "Caring about" International Patients in
   Delhi: Medical Travel Facilitation between Strategy
   and Sympathy ... 91
   Sarah Hartmann

6 Giving and Receiving Help across the Border: Transnational
   Health Practices of Migrants in Finland ... 115
   *Laura Kemppainen, Larisa Shpakovskaya, Inna Perheentupa,
   and Driss Habti*

7	The Dual Role of the Facilitator as Therapist and Reproductive Travel Broker in Cross-border Reproductive Travel from Developed Countries: Psychological and Ethical Perspectives and a Call for Separation of Services *Dr. Joyeeta G. Dastidar*	141
8	Complexity and Contradiction: Intimacy, Testimony, and Care in Humanitarian Aid *Elizabeth Lanphier*	155
9	The Invisible Work of Care and Emotions along the Trajectories of Beninese Children Traveling to Switzerland without Their Family for Heart Surgery *Carla Vaucher*	177

Index	201
About the Editor	203
About the Contributors	205

Exploring the Emotional Dimensions of Caring on the Move

An Introduction

Cecilia Vindrola-Padros

The use of travel to seek medical services in a nearby region and, even, a faraway country is currently common practice. An estimated 5 million people travel to obtain medical care in another country per year (Horsfall and Lunt 2016). Decisions to engage in medical travel are often shaped by the patients' and/or family members' desire to obtain cheaper or quicker services, treatments not available (or legal) near their home, or obtain culturally appropriate care (Vindrola-Padros et al. 2018). The process of traveling to obtain medical services has been referred to as medical travel, and this concept encompasses various forms of travel such as medical tourism, cross-border care, return migration, and more local forms of healthcare-related mobility (such as traveling within countries) (Vindrola-Padros 2019).

Traveling for care away from one's home is a complex process, involving multiple actors, a combination of journeys and careful planning. Those intending to travel need to obtain information about potential destinations and procedures, the best ways to get there, potential complications from the procedures or therapies, and arrangements for recovery (Crooks et al. 2017). In many cases, they also need to secure funding to cover the costs of travel and medical procedures (Bochaton 2015; Kangas 2007). They must also handle the logistics of traveling and being away from home, such as suspending employment, securing childcare, and making arrangements for caregivers who might be acting as companions during the journey or remaining at home (Vindrola-Padros et al. 2018).

All of these decisions to enable medical travel and the actual experience of traveling are imbued with the feelings and emotions of the traveler, companion, and all of those around them. As patients leave their place of origin, the caring duties of family members extend beyond local borders as they provide care to medical travelers on the move or take on new responsibilities in the place of origin (Kangas 2007). Global connectivity can change perceptions of the care available to patients, as they no longer need to restrict themselves to what is available locally (Kangas 2007). In a way, the possibility to travel to seek care elsewhere enacts feelings of hope as the chance of finding treatment, relief, or a cure are now plausible.

Emotional states prevalent during travel (i.e., wonder, anxiety, fear, excitement) are compounded by emotions associated with diagnosis (i.e., uncertainty) and treatment (i.e., hope), creating a complex web of feelings for those seeking and delivering care. Emotions guide decisions to seek care elsewhere, they influence the selection of destinations, shape the experience of care, and permeate stories of medical travel told to others upon return (Greco 2019). Emotions also guide the care work performed by professionals "tending the bodies of patients" (Ackerman 2010) as well as those who travel with patients who seek care elsewhere (Vindrola-Padros and Brage 2017). Medical travel brokers provide solace and comfort to anxious and worried patients (Speier 2011).

The role of caregivers (broadly defined) at home, during travel, and at the destination and how emotional states shape experiences and processes of medical travel remain unexplored areas of research (Casey et al. 2013a; Casey et al. 2013b; Crooks et al. 2017). The aim of this book is to shed light on the interconnections between caring, travel, and healthcare, placing an emphasis on the emotional dimensions of seeking care away from home.

The chapters in this volume explore the following questions:

- How do acts of curing, moving, and caring overlap?
- How is care work shaped by the need to move to other locations for medical services?
- How is travel configured and experienced by ill travelers who require care from family members or healthcare workers?
- What are the different layers of care involved in medical travel?
- How are processes of caring and care work conceptualized in cases where medical travel journeys are not physically enacted (but entail the flow of medication, advice and other types of information)?

The volume brings together contributions from a wide range of disciplines, including anthropology, nursing, primary care, sociology and geography, and covers experiences of medical travel and other forms of remote care in the United States, Laos, India, Italy, France, Finland, Switzerland, and Russia.

MEDICAL TRAVEL RESEARCH TODAY

Originally, the main patient flows explored in the medical travel literature were those of United States or European patients seeking elective care in the

Global South. Most of these studies did not focus on patients' experiences of care and were concerned with mapping the numbers of patients traveling abroad, trends in healthcare seeking, and identifying cases of complications (Burkett, 2007; Hunter & Oultram, 2010; Martin, 2010; Parks, 2010; Pennings, 2004; Storrow, 2005). More recent literature has shifted its focus to document the complex experiences of medical travelers and their interactions with healthcare systems and workers in their country of destination (Ackerman, 2010; Aizura, 2010; Bergmann, 2011; Edmonds, 2011; Green et al., 2016; Inhorn, 2008, 2015; Nolan, 2011; Song, 2010; Speier, 2016; Kangas, 2007, 2010; Vindrola-Padros, 2019; Whittaker, 2008).

Despite the widespread recognition of the complexity of medical travel, few studies have explored the arrangements that need to be put in place by traveling patients and their families to seek care elsewhere. Some authors have argued that medical travel is a highly burdensome process, entailing great physical and emotional labor (Kangas, 2007; 2010; Vindrola-Padros, 2011; 2012; 2019). A considerable gap in research is the exploration of the financial implications of medical travel (and how these expenses are normally covered), the arrangements that need to be made back home (i.e., employment, childcare, housework) as well as in the medical travel destination (i.e., accommodation, paperwork, other services). There is also a lack of research on the experiences of those accompanying medical travelers. Ethnographies on travel for pediatric oncology treatment (Brage, 2018; Vindrola-Padros, 2011, 2012) and Kangas' work (2007, 2010) have documented the role played by accompanying family members in facilitating journeys, coping with relocation and caring for family members who remained at home. This book takes a closer look at the caregiving role of travel companions (whether these are family members or healthcare workers) as well as instances when medical travelers care for themselves and take on the role of caregivers.

CARING AND EMOTIONS

Extensive work has been carried out to highlight the subjectivity engrained in medical thought and practice and the emotionally charged relationships that develop in medical encounters (Rapley 2008). These emotional states are further expanded when medical treatment requires some form of travel. The desire to experience particular emotions might be a trigger for movement, for instance, the desire to feel happiness or a sense of security through proximity with friends or relatives. Embodied states accompany movement, making those who travel experience their own sense of selfhood, purpose, and belonging (Lean et al., 2014). Destinations, places of origin, places in-between, and modes of transport will all create particular environments that stimulate the senses and create unique emotional states. Harvey and Knox (2012), for instance, argue that infrastructures, in the form of roads, have the capacity to generate a sense of enchantment, that is, a potential surprising encounter or unexpected events. Individuals might also experience multiple forms of ongoing emplacement, as in the case of migrants who continue to experience strong connections to their place of origin (Boellstorf & Linguist, 2004; Conradson & McKay, 2007; Davidson et al., 2005).

Emotions shape interactions and also "do work" in the sense that they create new meaning and might generate connections between individuals that did not exist before (White 2005). This emotional framing of experiences and interactions has also been studied in the context of organizations, including healthcare organizations, where organizational arrangements and cultures will appeal to the feelings of staff, will determine which emotions are allowed (or not) and how staff should respond to them (Hochschild 1983; Mann 1997). Staff working within organizations have the capacity to shape the emotion-work that they do, yet they can also experience a disconnection between the work performed and what they actually feel (Brighton et al. 2019; Pandey and Singh 2016). In the case of medical travel, this emotional work has been documented in the healthcare organizations where travelers obtain care, in the case of intermediaries who facilitate medical travel (i.e., medical travel facilitators) or those who provide non-clinical care to recovering patients (Ackerman et al. 2010; Dalstrom 2013; Hartmann 2019).

These processes of regulating and managing feelings, commonly referred to as emotional labor, require skills to respond to another person and their perceived needs, and identify the best way to address those needs (Hochschild 1983; James 1989; Smith 1992). Those skills are learned and can be refined over time (James 1992). Emotional labor is also gendered and shaped by ethnicity and social class, as some members of society perform this type of labor more frequently than others (England 2005; James 1992).

Emotional labor is inextricably linked to the concepts of care, caring, and care work. Care has been defined as the process of delivering sustained and close mental and physical attention to an individual (James 1992). Some authors have highlighted that instead of care, we should talk about "caring" to allude to its performative dimensions and the capacity of the individuals involved in the caring process to affect and be affected by another (Giraud and Hollin 2016). Caring should, therefore, be considered as an affective practice, as through acts of care individuals are produced as meaningful subjects. Care work brings to light acts of caring (physical and emotional) as a form of both paid and unpaid labor, labor that is recognized (valued and/or remunerated) as well as labor that remains invisible (England 2005). In the case of medical travel, some authors have argued that care work contributes to transnational connectivity, involving distant relationships and required instances of physical proximity (Kaspar and Reddy 2017).

ENGAGING WITH THIS BOOK

The chapters in this book provide insight into the psychological, emotional, cultural, political, and economic dimensions of caring on the move and at a distance. The authors use detailed case studies from around the world to explore how caring and care work are shaped by social situations as well as the space and time where/when caring takes place. Caring is also conceptualized as a dynamic concept, in continuous transformation, and shaped by the physical movement of those seeking and delivering care as well as the possibility of movement (even if the journey is never enacted).

The authors reflect on the caring roles of a wide range of actors, including instances when traveling patients care for themselves and others. In her study of the experiences of Beninese children seeking medical procedures in Switzerland as minors accompanied by non-governmental organization (NGO) volunteers (and no family members), Vaucher highlights the active role of child travelers in caring for themselves and other children traveling with them. She argues that the medical travel literature has underscored the role of some actors, such as surgeons, and rendered invisible the emotional work of others such as volunteers and traveling patients. In addition to providing physical care, children who shared their stories with her were able to manage their own emotions and those of others. Their agency was visible in clinical contexts and their experience of childhood on the move.

Crooks and Pickering highlight the role of family caregivers when travelers need to seek care abroad. In their analysis of the experiences of older Canadian couples who participate in international retirement migration in the United States, the authors document instances when one of the travelers has to access care abroad, highlighting the care work that needs to be performed by accompanying family members who are unpaid and untrained to carry out these tasks. The situation is further complicated by the fact that many of these caregivers do not see themselves as such (and do not access caregiving support) and also have care needs of their own.

Other dominant actors that appear in the chapters are medical travel facilitators (MTFs), that is, organizations, companies, or individuals who facilitate the travel of patients to another location to obtain medical treatment. Hartmann considers MTFs as her object of study to explore the negotiation of caring in a commercial context. According to her, the care work of MTFs includes dimensions of "caring for" (ensuring material and general well-being) and "caring about" (emotional aspects of caring and a sense of attachment to traveling patients and their families) that cannot be disentangled. As international patients are considered both social and economic actors, their caring will undoubtedly comprise practices of care as a business strategy and humane actions. Dastidar continues this conversation regarding the role of these intermediaries asking if there is a conflict relating to how much facilitators should do. Is there a limit to their caring? Are boundaries transgressed due to the uniqueness of the context of delivering/receiving care away from home? Dastidar engages in a critical discussion of the expectations regarding the role of these intermediaries, but highlights that standards have not been developed at an international scale to validate their practices and few MTFs are provided with training opportunities.

Dalstrom takes the discussion of the role of MTFs facilitating medical travel journeys of U.S. patients to Mexico in a different direction by using these experiences to examine the limitations of the U.S. healthcare system. According to him, medical travel experiences (the reasons why patients need to seek care abroad and what they liked about these services) can be used to improve healthcare in the United States, delivering more personalized care, support that extends beyond the clinical encounter, and time and close, empathic, relationships with care providers. Greco, as she documents the journeys of patients with breast cancer in Italy and France, identifies a similar overlap between what she refers to as the logics of care and cure. The women seeking care in her chapter made decisions to travel to obtain what they considered to be higher quality care than what was available locally. Quality meant different things to the women and patient choices were shaped by feelings of trust, affection, and the attentiveness of care providers.

Feelings of trust take on a central role in the chapter by Kemppainen and colleagues, where the authors explore the creation of transnational therapy networks spanning actors in Finland and Russia with the aim of sharing healthcare information, advice, and medications. Trust in others who speak a similar language and are able to share a common therapeutic experience is the reason to develop and make use of these networks. The chapter demonstrates that medical travel and caring do not always entail acts of physical movement or proximity as both can also be facilitated through virtual landscapes.

The chapters contribute to the unpacking of caring processes, highlighting instances when caring might imply closer connections through intimacy as well as episodes of detachment. In her analysis of the first personal accounts of humanitarian aid workers, Lanphier shifts our attention from those receiving care to those delivering it and proposes that care involves intertwined dimensions of abstraction and intimacy. She urges us to consider humanitarian aid workers as situated beings with affective attachments that generate internal tensions when, in order to care for others far from home, they must distance themselves from their traditional caring relationships. Furthermore, caring roles in humanitarian contexts are complex as those caring for others can easily become those being cared for (as in the case of local staff caring for expatriates).

Some authors use the concept of reciprocity as a lens to explore caring relationships. Lanphier argues that reciprocity and mutuality are not requirements for the delivery of care, as care can be provided to others without expecting anything in return. Thao and Bochaton, in their exploration of the experiences of Hmong Americans who engage in the circulation of care with networks in Laos to obtain access to herbal medicines, argue that an "economy of reciprocity" brings together transnational family networks. According to the authors, care circulation entails the "reciprocal, multidirectional and asymmetrical exchange of care" with the purpose of accessing a specific type of care that Hmong Americans cannot access in their place of origin, care that goes beyond the treatment of the individual body.

In one way or another, most of the chapters in the book also provide a critical analysis of medical travel, not seeing it as a process enacted by a "patient-consumer" (Ormond 2013) who makes rational decisions to seek care elsewhere (because it is cheaper, quicker or better), but understanding medical travel as a complex process produced by local and global inequalities in access to care. Dalstrom and Kemppainen and colleagues draw from Castaneda's (2018) concept of migrants being "stuck in motion" in the sense that their need to seek medical services away from home is produced by the local barriers they face accessing care in their place of residence. Dalstrom encourages us to ask ourselves, who has the capacity to move? Who can order high-cost drugs and receive care in a private clinic? Vaucher also contributes to this discussion by reflecting on the experiences of travel of ill children from a low income country who seek care in a high income country. She argues that their life-saving journeys are cross-cut by prolonged family separation and profound emotional situations for children who travel without close family members and parents who stay at home and place their trust in volunteers and a dream of medical cure in a distant country. Would those experiences be different if the same procedure was performed close to home?

Some of the chapters in the book argue that additional research is required to capture the nuances of caring and care work in the context of medical travel. This book represents a starting point, but we need to continue to explore caring and caregiving in practice, its multiple dimensions, and contradictions. This will entail continuing to unpack what we mean by caring and care work, how these concepts change over time and during movement, and discovering hidden forms of care work and emotional labor, and carers who have remained invisible until now.

We will also need to explore caring and medical travel in the context of a new global landscape. As this book was being developed the world was actively struggling with the management of the COVID-19 pandemic. The pandemic shaped the experiences of the authors who, in the face of new pressures and uncertainty, carried on to put together engaging and insightful chapters. The pandemic has also shaped current and future forms of medical travel that will need to be studied in detail. As new restrictions for physical movement have emerged, how have those desiring/needing care away from home coped? Have ideas of what constitutes medical travel (and caring) changed as a result? Have global provider networks adapted to deliver care in a different way? These questions will pave the way for a new area of inquiry in a field of medical travel shaped by global pandemics, climate change, telemedicine and remote monitoring, and profound transformations in our way of seeing transport and travel.

REFERENCES

Ackerman, S. 2010. "Plastic paradise: Transforming bodies and selves in Costa Rica's cosmetic surgery tourism industry." *Medical Anthropology* 29(4), 403–423.

Aizura, Aren 2010. "Feminine transformations: Gender reassignment surgical tourism in Thailand." *Medical Anthropology* 29(4), 424–443.

Bergmann, S. 2011. "Fertility tourism: Circumventive routes that enable access to reproductive technologies and substances." *Signs* 36(2), 280–289.

Bochaton, Audrey. 2015. "Cross-border mobility and social networks: Laotians seeking medical treatment along the Thai border." *Social Science & Medicine* 124, 364–373.

Boellstorff, T., and Lindquist, J. 2004. "Bodies of emotion: Rethinking culture and emotion through Southeast Asia." *Ethnos* 69(4), 437–444.

Brage, E. 2018. "Si no fuera porque me vine...". Itinerarios terapéuticos y prácticas de cuidado en el marco de las migraciones desarrolladas desde el Noroeste y Noreste Argentino hacia la Ciudad Autónoma de Buenos Aires para la atención del cáncer infantil: Un abordaje antropológico. Tesis doctoral. Facultad de Filosofía y Letras, Universidad de Buenos Aires.

Burkett, L. 2007. "Medical tourism: Concerns, benefits, and the American legal perspective." *The Journal of Legal Medicine* 28, 223–245.

Casey, V., Crooks, V.A., Snyder, J., and Turner, L. 2013a. "Knowledge brokers, companions, and navigators: a qualitative examination of informal caregivers' roles in medical tourism." *Int J Equity Health* 12:94.

Casey, V., Crooks, V.A., Snyder, J., Turner, L. 2013b. "You're dealing with an emotionally charged individual...": an industry perspective on the challenges posed by medical tourists' informal caregiver-companions." *Global Health* 9:31.

Castañeda, H. 2018. 'Stuck in Motion': Simultaneous Mobility and Immobility in Migrant Healthcare Along the US-Mexico Border. *Healthcare in Motion: Immobilities in Health Service Delivery and Access*, Vindrola-Padros, C., G. Johnson and A. Pfister, eds. 19–34. Berghahn Books: UK.

Conradson, D., McKay, D. 2007. "Translocal subjectivities: Mobility, connection, emotion." *Mobilities* 2(2), 167–174.

Crooks, V.A., Whitmore, R., Snyder, J., Turner, L. 2017. "Ensure that you are well aware of the risks you are taking...": actions and activities medical tourists' informal caregivers can undertake to protect their health and safety. *BMC Public Health* 17(1):487.

Dalstrom, Matthew. 2013. "Medical travel facilitators: connecting patients and providers in a globalized world." *Anthropology & Medicine* 20, no. 1, 24–35.

Davidson, J., Bondi, L., Smith, M. 2005. *Emotional geographies*. Aldershot: Ashgate.

Edmonds, A. 2011. "Almost invisible scars: Medical tourism to Brazil." *Signs* 36(2), 297–302.

England, Paula. 2005. "Emerging theories of care work." *Annu. Rev. Sociol.* 31: 381–399.

Giraud, Eva, Hollin, G. 2016. "Care, Laboratory Beagles and Affective Utopia." *Theory, Culture & Society* 33(4): 27–49.

Greco, Cinzia. 2019. "Moving for cures: Breast cancer and mobility in Italy." *Medical Anthropology* 38, no. 4: 384–398.

Green, S. (2013). "Borders and the relocation of Europe." *Annual Review of Anthropology*, 42, 345–361.

Hartmann, Sarah. 2019. "Mobilising patients towards transnational healthcare markets–insights into the mobilising work of medical travel facilitators in Delhi." *Mobilities* 14, no. 1 (2019): 71–86.

Harvey, P., Knox, H. 2012. "The enchantments of infrastructure." *Mobilities* 7(4), 521–536.

Hochschild, A.R. 1983. *The Managed Heart: Commercialization of Human Feeling*. Berkeley: Univ. Calif. Press

Horsfall, D., Lunt, N. 2016. Medical tourism by numbers. In: Handbook on medical tourism and patient mobility, edited by N. Lunt, D. Horsfall, and J. Hanefled, 25–36. Cheltenham, UK: Edward Elgar.

Hunter, D., Oultram, S. 2010. "The ethical and policy implications of rogue medical tourism." *Global Social Policy* 10, 297–299

Inhorn, M. 2007. "Masculinity, reproduction and male infertility surgeries in Egypt and Lebanon." *Journal of Middle East Women's Studies* 3(3), 1–20.

Inhorn, M. 2015. *Cosmopolitan conceptions: IVF sojourns in global Dubai*. Durham: Duke University Press.

James, N. 1989. "Emotional labour." *Sociological Review* 37, 15–42.

James, N. 1992. "Care organisation and physical labour and emotional." *Soc Health Ill* 14, 4.

Kangas, B. 2007. "Hope from abroad in the international medical travel of Yemeni patients." *Anthropology and Medicine* 14(3), 293–305.

Kangas, B. 2011. "Complicating common ideas about medical tourism: Gender, class, and globality in Yemeni's international medical travel." *Signs* 36(2), 327–332.

Kaspar, Heidi, Reddy, S. 2017. "Spaces of connectivity: The formation of medical travel destinations in Delhi National Capital Region (India)." *Asia Pacific Viewpoint* 58, no. 2: 228–241.

Lean, G., Staiff, R., Waterton, E. 2014. *Travel and imagination*. Farnham: Ashgate.
Mann, S. 1997. "Emotional labour in organizations." *Leadership & Organization Development Journal* 18 (1): 4–12.
Martin, D. 2010. "Ethical issues in medical travel for human biological materials." *Global Social Policy*, 10, 3.
Mol, A. 2008. *The logic of care: Health and the problem of patient choice*. London: Routledge.
Nolan, J. M., Schneider, M. J. 2011. "Medical tourism in the backcountry: Alternative health and healing in the Arkansas Ozarks." *Signs* 36(2), 319–326.
Ormond, Meghann. 2013. *Neoliberal governance and international medical travel in Malaysia*. Vol. 9. Routledge.
Parks, J. 2010. "Care ethics and the global practice of commercial surrogacy." *Bioethics* 24, 323–332.
Pennings, G. 2004. "Legal harmonization and reproductive tourism in Europe." *Human Reproduction* 19, 2689–2694.
Rapley, Tim. 2008. "Distributed Decision Making: The Anatomy of Decisions-in-Action." *Sociology of Health & Illness* 30(3): 141–9889.
Smith, P. 1992. *The Emotional Labour of Nursing*. Basingstoke: Macmillan.
Song, P. 2010. "Biotech pilgrims and the transnational quest for stem cell cures." *Medical Anthropology* 29(4), 384–402.
Speier, A. 2011. "Brokers, consumers and the Internet: How North American consumers navigate their infertility journeys." *Reproductive Biomedicine Online* 23(5), 592–599.
Speier, A. 2016. *Fertility holidays: IVF tourism and the reproduction of whiteness*. New York: New York University Press.
Storrow, R. 2005. "Quests for conception: Fertility tourists, globalization and feminist legal theory." *Hastings Legal Journal* 57, 295–330.
Vindrola-Padros, C. 2011. *Life and death journeys: medical travel, cancer and children in Argentina*. PhD. Department of Anthropology, University of South Florida.
Vindrola-Padros, C. 2019. *Critical ethnographic perspectives on medical travel*. London: Routledge.
Vindrola-Padros, C., Brage, E. 2017. Child medical travel in Argentina: Narratives of family separation and moving away from home. In C. R. Ergler & R. A. Kearnes (Eds.), Children's health and wellbeing in urban environments. London: UK: Routledge.
Vindrola-Padros, C., Brage, E., Chambers, P. 2018. "On the road and away from home: a systematic review of the travel experiences of cancer patients and their families." *Supportive Care in Cancer* 26, 2973–2982.
Whittaker, A. 2008. "Pleasure and pain: medical travel in Asia." *Global Public Health* 3(3), 271–290.

Chapter 1

Healing in the Diaspora

Hmong American and Hmong Lao Practices of Care

Mai See Thao and Audrey Bochaton

There was an old man [Hmong American] who was supposed to die within a week and he came here [Laos] and drank a lot of Hmong green herbs. Some come here for *tshuaj tshuab* (green herbs) and ask around with their relatives for herbs. It's sometimes $100 and these are *tshuaj hav zoo* (medicine from the forest). They have to use their *tswv yim* (wisdom) when American medicine fails them.

(Bee Thao, Vientiane, Laos)

In the dry season, I sometimes go and gather plants myself, but only those that I can find around my home. Otherwise, I order large quantities of plants from many pickers in the surrounding villages, especially during the rainy season, when picking conditions are difficult. I also sometimes order from Hmong relatives in Vietnam who bring me plants that cannot be found in Laos. For shipments to the United States, I mainly ship mixtures of dried plants and chopped roots. My youngest daughter and daughter-in-law help me condition the plants and prepare labels with therapeutic indications and how to prepare them. For the American market, I sell mainly for lung, heart, kidney problems and also for hypertension, diabetes and obesity problems.

(Pa Shoua Her, Tham Say village, Nong Het district, Laos)

The movement of bodies and herbs in the Hmong diaspora[1] is a circulation of care that transcends the nation-state boundaries of Laos and the United States. These circulations reconnect Hmong Lao and Hmong Americans to their once-distant union and offer up new possibilities through its frictions (Tsing 2005). In this chapter, we draw on Loretta Baldassar and Laura Merla's (2014) definition of care circulation as "the reciprocal, multidirectional and asymmetrical exchange of care that fluctuates over the life course within transnational family networks subject to the political, economic, cultural and social contexts of both sending and receiving societies" (p. 22). Those who seek care in Laos and consume the herbal medicines from Laos are Hmong Americans who are first-generation refugees, having left Laos either as a young adult or child after 1975. Having aged in the United States and developed chronic diseases, Hmong Americans return to Laos for the hopes of care beyond the biomedical care that treats just the individual and somatic body (Thao MS 2018a). These circulations, which allow Hmong Americans to reassert and soothe their ailment in context, are embedded in a long-standing colonial history and geopolitics in Southeast Asia. Indeed, understanding these transnational circulations of care requires studying the broader historical background of Hmong displacement from the history of French colonialism to American imperialism in Southeast Asia.

Laos was colonized by the French from 1893 to 1945 and during the height of the Cold War between the United States and USSR (1954), the French were defeated by the Viet Minh communist revolutionaries and consequently, relinquished control of their colonies in Indochina (Vietnam, Laos, and Cambodia). Despite the 1954 Geneva Accords that declared Laos as neutral, the United States and North Vietnam (USSR's proxy) meddled in Lao politics, furthering divisions within the country. Violating the Geneva Accords, the U.S. Central Intelligence Agency (CIA) sought out Hmong General Vang Pao to recruit Hmong and other Lao ethnic minorities to fight a proxy war on behalf of the United States in the eastern regions of Laos against the Communist Pathet Lao and the North Vietnamese Army. It is estimated that 17,000 Hmong died in the war (Hamilton-Merritt 1993). As casualties swelled, the fighting transitioned to air warfare. The United States dropped 2 million tons of bombs in Laos alone, the most in the history of the world (Chan 1991). This war would not be made public to Americans until 1969 when the United States was already looking to exit the war in Southeast Asia (Chan 1994). Due to its secrecy from the American public and Congress, this war in Laos is known as the Secret War.

Putting an end to the Vietnam War, a ceasefire was signed at the Paris Peace Accords on January 1973. Many Hmong soldiers felt "used and abandoned" by their American allies (Hamilton-Merrit 1993; Lee M 2018). In Laos, the communist Pathet Lao took over the government in 1975. Some

Hmong families sought to return back to their lives in Laos, but the increasing reprisal of the Pathet Lao against those who fought with the Americans made Laos increasingly dangerous for the Hmong. In 1980, 102,479 refugees, 95 percent of whom were Hmong, arrived in camps in Thailand (Stuart-Fox 1997; Vang CY 2010). It is estimated that 150,000 Hmong left Laos (Chan 1994).

Hmong resettlement in the United States was not granted until December of 1975 (Hillmer 2010). They were relocated to the United States, France, Australia, Germany, and French Guiana. In the United States, the Hmong were first dispersed throughout the nation to avoid over-burdening states, only to result in a secondary migration where Hmong later chose to migrate to places where their families lived to make cultural adjustment easier (Chan 1991). This secondary migration gave way to Hmong mostly residing in California, Minnesota, and Wisconsin.

While some Hmong refugees resettled in the United States, some of their family members remained in Laos. Those who chose to stay in Laos sought to return to their normal life, some sympathized with the Communist Party (Lee M. 2015), and about 15,000 of General Vang Pao's followers retreated in the jungles and continued to wage resistance against the Laotian government (Lee G., 1982). This rupture within Hmong kinship and the Hmong community paves way for the transnational circulation of Hmong products and commodities such as food, clothing, and cultural objects across the Mekong Region (Yun 2010) and beyond (Culhane-Pera et al. 2003). We will explore in particular the circulation of medicinal herbs and the return of Hmong American bodies to Laos for health and healing and the affect that these practices are caught within.

In this chapter, we examine the possibilities and politics of hope, love, and its messiness within the transnational circulation of care which is beyond the treatment of just the body and the consumption of herbs. We draw on Judith B. Farquhar's (1994) attention to the pleasures of medicine. Rather than to see the consumption of herbal medicines and returns to Laos as just a means to health, we examine the affective and political components of care in this transnational circulation. We examine the pleasures of care in consuming herbal medicine from the mountains of Laos, the family network that is activated and maintained in the travel of Hmong herbal healers from Laos as well as the transfer of advice through telephone calls and internet (Bochaton 2018), the ways the return of the Hmong American body is reconnected with displaced family members, and the participation of family in the effort to find a cure and care for Hmong American aliments (Thao MS 2018a).

In this chapter, our fieldwork shows that transnational cares is a form of messy care work. Indeed the pleasures caught up in Hmong transnational cares is gendered care work (Hondagneu-Sotelo 2001), where mostly women constitute those sending herbs and sources of affection, but not always. As well, the movement of bodies to Laos and the sending of herbs from Laos to the United States draws on Third World labor (Horschild 2000). The commodification of transnational cares also allows Hmong Lao access to economic mobility not possible in Laos (England & Folbre 2000), rejecting "the idea of an oppositional dichotomy between the realms of love and self-interested economic action" (England 2005, 392). However, the affects of Hmong familial love and hope queers care work. Familial love and hope structures a homogenous Hmong community beyond normative practices of patriarchy, gender, and ethno-national formations of community[2]. It revises long histories of ethnic and national histories of conflict and tension and troubles economic explanation of care work by creating an economy of reciprocity that sutures and maintains the disrupted familial relationships in the diaspora. Therefore, we describe our work as a transnational circulation of care to insist on its reciprocity or perhaps, indebtedness.[3] That is not to say these potentialities overcomes the tensions and ambivalences of care work nor the divergent histories of the Hmong diaspora noted earlier.

This chapter asks: How does the medical travel of plants, humans, and kinship reconstitute a displaced community? How are the processes of transnational caring, as care work, shaped by the cultural, historical, social, and political characteristics of Hmong diaspora? While migration for care can be hopeful, we ask why does care also entails ambivalence? In answering these questions, we draw on both of our fieldwork from Laos; one multi-sited ethnography carried out in Hmong herbal medicine markets in Laos (Bochaton 2010–2011) and consisting of interviews with traditional healers, with plants sellers, and pickers in different villages; another multi-sited ethnography investigated sites of returns for health and healing for Hmong Americans that included visiting herbalist and consuming Hmong herbs in Laos (Thao 2014–2015).

PLEASURES OF CARE AND THERAPEUTIC LANDSCAPES: QUEST FOR TRANSNATIONAL HEALING

In Dr. Thao's work (2018a) on Hmong American with type 2 diabetes, Hmong Americans articulate *kev nyuaj siab*, literally translated as the "path" (*kev*) of the "difficult liver" (*nyuaj siab*) as the largest contributor to their diabetes experiences. Unlike the heart in American cultural understandings of emotion, the liver is the seat of emotion for the Hmong. It encompasses the "full gamut of experience, thought, emotion, and sensation as well as the processes of daily life such as talking" (Henry 1996, 23). Moreover, the expression *kev nyuaj siab* points to a large social and historical context that is missed in the biomedical translation of depression.[4] Dr. Thao comprehends "the path of the difficult liver" as rooted in a larger Hmong American experience of displacement in the United States, from the Secret War to the trauma of resettlement in the United States to ongoing structured experiences of displacement in biomedicine and the United States' changing labor markets.

This chapter's theoretical framework expands on Dr. Thao's work on the liver to understand how the pleasures in returning to Laos for healing and the consumption of Hmong herbal medicines work to soothe the difficult liver. The soothing qualities of these practices are hope and love as detailed later. However, we use the term soothing to also imply that these pleasures are temporary. They are also ambivalent, entangled within the frictions of globalizations (Tsing 2005) and Hmong American and Hmong Lao historical tensions.

Soothing is an intentional term we employ to understand the multiple ways the liver is soothed through the familial and commercial care works, the engagement and embodiment of Laos's therapeutic landscapes (Gesler 1992), and the consumption of Hmong herbal medicines. In order to first understand how these herbs and returns are soothing/healing, it is important to begin on a foundation that moves beyond biomedical functionalist ideas of medicine, such as the preoccupation with whether these herbs and returns truly *cure* people. For example, a functionalist question would be "Do their A1c (blood glucose levels) decrease while in Laos?" or "Does their diabetes really get better?" Situating these diasporic engagements beyond a biomedical means-to-ends model, reveals the ways affect like hope and love, caught within returns and Hmong herbal consumption, can form the transnational circulation of care we describe.

Van der Geest and Whyte (1989) argue that with the commodification of medicines and their movement, they move as objects that carry metonymic associations. In their case on pharmaceutical medicines, the knowledge of doctors and their technological expertise are carried within the pharmaceutical medicines as things-in-themselves. The context that produces the medicines is the value that is transactional in the commodification and circulation of medicines. In the circulation of Hmong herbal medicines and the returns of Hmong Americans to Laos for healing, plants from Laotian mountains and the country itself offer up hope for Hmong Americans who are the largest consumers of this circulation of care. As this chapter will show, Hmong herbs carry the essence of Hmongness. Hmong herbal medicines and sites of returns are constructed and seen to embody characters of Hmongness as "natural" and "green" and in opposition to the "artificialness" of Western medicine. Hmong herbs are seen to not have the same side effects as Western medicine because they carry with them the essence of Hmongness, naturalness (Culhane-Pera et al 2007). They and Laos are articulated as "made" for Hmong bodies whereas biomedical medicines are made for white American bodies.

The social contexts of where these herbs originate in Laos and the social construction of these herbs as inherently Hmong, builds on Gesler's concept of "therapeutic landscape" (1992). Therapeutic landscape brings together the notion of a landscape with principles of holistic health and has been applied to a wide range of places, settings, situations, and contexts that encompass both the physical and psychological environments associated with treatment or healing, and the maintenance of health and well-being. Gesler's early work was concerned with physical locations considered to be beneficial to physical, mental, and spiritual healing and well-being in health settings such as Lourdes, France and Bath, England (William 1998, Perriam 2015). Since then, the concept has evolved to consider more diverse and holistic relationships between health and the environment and has been applied in health geography and health anthropology. According to William (2007), therapeutic landscapes gather formal therapeutic sites such as healthcare institutions as well as informal therapeutic sites where work on the self or where improvement to subjective well-being may take place. We use "therapeutic landscapes" to understand how the sites of herbal treatments, herbal cultivation, and the mountainous landscapes of Laos work as informal or symbolic sites which are therapeutic in two ways: they contain both the aesthetics of the original space (Odgen 2015) and the plants used for traditional remedies in the Hmong community. When the plants are purchased on the urban markets in Laos or in the United States, then carefully prepared and finally absorbed, they embody at all stages the landscapes of Laos and work as a memory of what it means to be Hmong. The mobility of bodies and herbs are therapeutic in the ways it calls upon the various affective attributes of the liver (of consumption/ingestion/herbal sensations, experience of being in their old country, and to reviving a past youthful self).

The movement of these herbs and bodies across space and time are also more than just appealing and desirable. "Transnational configurations of medicine and health have led to the production and articulation of subjectivities, desires, and intimacies which are imagined and articulated in and through the flows of people, technologies and resources across national and continental borders" (Dilger, Kane, Langwick 2012 p. 15). Reconnecting displaced family members in the diaspora, these forms of cares ultimately soothes what was displaced (Hmong identity and community). Its circulation works to structure and maintain a reciprocal economy of care for the Hmong diaspora, indebting Hmong Americans to Hmong Lao. And yet, soothing highlights its ephemeral qualities. Transnational cares are situated within social, historical, and political contexts that give way to tensions and issues of power within the Hmong diaspora. Offering up hope and love to soothe a larger Hmong American displacement, these cares are ultimately ambivalent. They are haunted by the historical divisions within the Hmong diaspora that date the time of French colonialism, the memory of Hmong American departure from Laos, Hmong American returns as the extension of American imperialism, and the frictions of hope and love as commodity within the intimate spaces of familial love and community. This chapter draws on the practices of soothing the "difficult liver" to understand the appeal and power within transnational cares among Hmong community.

Method

This chapter weaves together two fieldworks from Drs. Bochaton (2011) and Thao (2014–2015). All names used in this chapter are pseudonyms. Dr. Bochaton's investigations focus on data collection in Xiengkouang province in the north-east of Laos, specifically in Phonsavan and Nong Het district, a mountainous and remote area along the border with Vietnam. The data were gathered by ethnographic methods and consists of interviews with traditional healers, with plants sellers, and pickers in different villages. Records from the Lao Post Office were also collected as they contain information concerning the content and value of packages sent abroad. Finally in March 2012, Bochaton had the opportunity to visit and to have informal discussion with vendors of medicinal plants in a Hmong market in Saint Paul, United States.

Dr. Thao's fieldwork is also a multi-sited ethnographic study that examined why Hmong Americans with type 2 diabetes were engaging in returns for health and healing in Laos. While informed by her fieldwork and interviews conducted in a primary care clinic and interviews with Hmong Americans with type 2 diabetes in Saint Paul, MN, this chapter draws on ethnographic data from Thaos' six months of fieldwork (2014–2015) in Laos that followed the routes of returns for Hmong Americans in Laos. Following the recommendations of her Hmong American interviewees, Dr. Thao traveled to Vientiane, Xieng Khouang, and Luang Prabang. She conducted in-depth interviews with Hmong Lao about the returns of their family members from the United States, participant-observation of Hmong American returnees and their engagement with Hmong traditional herbs, and attending markets with Hmong Lao herbalist and interviewing herbalists about the sale of herbs to Hmong Americans.

HOPE: BEYOND BIOMEDICINE'S COLONIAL PAST AND PRESENT

"Medical capabilities existing abroad provided hope when local medical services could offer little. A doctor explained that families might send incurable cases abroad, 'because hope does not die.' Another doctor stated: 'Although the case is incurable, there still remains some hope for the patient and his family. Even if it is very small, they search for it no matter where.' Still another doctor referred to a proverb: 'The perplexed holds onto any tree'." (Kangas 2007)

The hope of pursuing treatment abroad generally refers to transnational patients looking for an advanced, trustworthy technological medicine that is unavailable locally. In our case study, the configuration is reversed. Hmong Americans going to Laos or receiving care from Laos are not seeking more technologically advanced medicine. Instead, the transnational circulation of care offers up the hopes of a return to a landscape in Laos that is deemed inherently Hmong and "traditional" forms of care. In the literature, there are other examples of return medical travels in order to access traditional care in the origin country. According to Tiilikainen (2012), Somali diaspora living in Finland and different European countries return to Somaliland in order to visit mostly traditional healers. Kane (2012) shows as well how Senegalese migrants based in France (the Haalpulaar community) choose to return back to Senegal for healthcare as they believe that certain types of illnesses like chronic diseases cannot be healed by Western medicine and that traditional or religious forms of healing are more appropriate. In our case study, these forms of cares also provide a critique against the colonial and imperial historical context of medicine for Hmong Americans.

"Hmong must use their *twv yim* (wisdom) when American medicine fails them" is a statement situated within a larger French colonial and U.S. imperial context. In Laos, Hmong lived in remote areas with little access to Western-trained health care providers and Western medicine until the USAID-sponsored medical relief efforts were established in the 1960s (Weldon, 1999). Before this period, although public health was considered a pillar of the "civilizing mission" during the French protectorate from 1893 to 1954 (Mignot, 2003), the health policy developed by the French was actually very limited due to of the country's isolation, low human densities, and the lower frequency of serious epidemics (cholera, tuberculosis) in comparison with current Vietnam and Cambodia (Ibid). Most dispensaries (37 in 1926) were concentrated in the most accessible areas of the Mekong plains, mainly in the provinces of Vientiane, Luang Prabang, Thakhek, Savannakhet, and Pakse. They, therefore, mainly targeted the Thai Lao populations and very little the mountain populations of which the Hmong are a part.

After the French dissolved their rule of Indochina in 1954, the United States continued to partially fund Laos, particularly in education, and increased their funds as the American War continued in Laos. Dr. Charles Weldon, who oversaw the Public Health Division of USAID in Laos, administered the Village Health Program which recruited the first Hmong nurse, Choua Thao. He often used colonial discourse to describe Lao ethnic nurses as children, writing about Choua as "girl" and her husband a "boy" despite them having two children in his diary (Vang CY 2016, pg. 64, 67). Despite the racialized and unequal treatment that Choua faced compared to her white counterpart, Diana (Dee) Quill, Choua and her team of two Mein, two Lao, two Lao Theung, and one Tai Dam cared for 8,500 people who fled enemy attack through the jungles, cared for villagers and wounded soldiers, and recruited and trained more nurses as the war continued on. Choua and Diana trained illiterate young women to employ American medications, teaching them basic nursing skills such as intravenous techniques, where 3,500 became health workers. Another Hmong woman, at the age of twelve years old, was recruited by the hospital in Sam Thong where she and others were trained "from surgery to pharmacy to labor delivery room" (Vang CY 2016, p. 69). She spent most of her time in the emergency room and delivery room in Long Cheng, the military base of the Hmong General Vang Pao (Vang CY 2016).

Hmong who fled from Laos after 1975 would also encounter allopathic medicine in the Thai refugee camps in the 1970s and 1980s (Wright 1986). Hmong people had mixed reactions to Western medicine within these settings; "They were impressed with the efficacy of intravenous fluids, blood transfusions, antibiotics, and operations that repaired war wounds. But they also were concerned about the adverse effects of Western therapies" (Culhane-Pera et al. 2003). Unlike the prestige and financial reward for Hmong parents who had Hmong daughters trained as nurses during the war (Vang CY 2016), Hmong refugees were wary of physicians' (mainly Thai and foreigners) procedures and motives in the camps: religious proselytizing was connected with health care, and Hmong refugees associated deaths and medical complications with the unfamiliar healthcare practices (Wright 1986). Some of them assumed that improper medicines were being given to them.

Encounters with medicine upon resettlement in the United States was described by journalist Anne Fadiman as a "culture shock" for both Hmong refugees and their white American doctors. In her book, *The Spirit Catches You and You Fall Down,* the "cultural shock" was attributed to differing perceptions of appropriate health treatment procedures (Fadiman 1998; Dia 2003). However, this lens never situated Hmong within larger issues of power (Taylor 2003a). Fadiman racializes the Hmong in the United States as hypervisibly cultural (Pha 2017), primitive, and existing out of time (Vang M 2012,

Thao 2018b). Hmong seeking medical care were often the subject of medical racism (Chiu 2004) and also experienced structural inequalities especially around language (Thao 2018b). Hmong refugees too were aware of biomedicine as also "cultural knowledge" (Taylor 2003b), informed and situated within U.S. racial and social politics (Thao 2018a). For example, in Thao's work on diabetes (2018a), Hmong Americans with type 2 diabetes articulate that doctors treat the individual body by focusing on biological values such as blood glucose, weight, and blood pressure. Hmong American diabetics articulated the need to treat the larger context of diabetes, the malady of being displaced persons in the United States and its embodiment.

Hmong Americans transgress the limits of biomedicine by drawing up hope for healing that resides beyond Western conceptualizations of health and healing. They seek forms of care that attend to the embodiment of a Hmong displacement. Hmong chronic diseases embody the ongoing legacy of imperialism in their post-refugee lives in a racialized capitalistic nation-state. Living in the empire, Hmong Americans continue to experience the unraveling of communal ties, cultural dislocation, loss of self-worth, the continual displacement of economic jobs, and economic precarity. These forms of displacement are somaticized and exacerbate chronic diseases (Thao 2019). Therefore, the pleasures and therapeutics of consuming and returning to places of familiarity offer up the hopes of addressing this aliment. Hmong medicine and Hmong returns offer up soothing qualities of a return, consumption, and practice involved in the essence of Hmongness that was displaced.

The Hopes of Hmong Herbal Medicine

Hmong therapies of healings and medicinal herbal uses have persisted in the United States despite war, displacement, and resettlement. Fleeing Laos, Hmong medicines were an important object to carry. Hmong refugees carried their collections of plants on the long journey from the northern highlands of Laos to the lowland refugee camps in Thailand. However, the amount of plants was low because of the heat and of the long distance covered on foot. Medicinal herbal knowledge is actively practiced especially among older Hmong. "Use of traditional herbal medicine has remained part of the world of Hmong women in the United States, where gifted elders have continued to teach female relatives and trusted friends" (Corlett et al. 2003).

In the United States, Hmong American women continue to grow Hmong medicine, mostly growing plants in summer gardens or in winter greenhouses. In Sacramento (California), for example, "the Hmong continue their agrarian traditions by creating urban gardens where they grow traditional plants either for food or medicinal use" (Corlett et al. 2003). But, as tropical plants can be difficult to obtain or to grow, exchange and trade networks exist within the American Hmong community: for example, they send fresh plants from warmer to colder parts of the country. Nevertheless, some herbs cannot be grown anywhere in the United States, which makes the continuation of traditional herbal healings difficult. This "lack of familiar plants has led to the importation of traditional Hmong herbs to California whether through covert commercial exchange or through covert personal transportation" (Corlett et al 2003, 366). In her work tracking Hmong herbal circulation out from Laos, Dr. Bochaton (2018) found that the United States, particularly the city of Saint Paul, Minnesota, received the majority of Hmong herbal shipments. Ranking behind St. Paul are U.S. cities Fresno and Sacramento, California.

Hmong herbal medicine is often categorized as "traditional Hmong medicine." In this chapter, we call them Hmong herbal medicines or *tshuaj tshuab* (green herbs) or *tshauj hav zoo* (herbs/medicine from the jungle) as Hmong themselves identify them as. These medicines are defined as inherently Hmong and often cultivated from the jungles, away from the modernity of chemical fertilizers and mass production. Knowledge of these medicines are apprenticed from other herbalists or Hmong herbalists are also informed by their spirit guides (*dab tshuaj/dab neeb*—similar to Shamans) that lead them to herbs that can heal ailments. During Dr. Thao's ethnographic fieldwork, Hmong herbalists agreed that Laos has the strongest Hmong herbal medicines, especially in the region of Nong Het. Dr. Bochaton's findings also support these claims as the majority of Hmong medicine shipped from Laos to the Hmong American consumers in the United States are from Nong Het.

As Dr. Thao (2018a) argues, this historical region has social, historical, and political valence, as it was an area of Hmong momentary autonomy. During French colonization of Laos, two Hmong leaders Touby Lyfong and Lo Fay Dang emerged, under French legitimation, to control Nong Het. During the Indochina War, the French appointed Touby Lyfong as district governor of Xieng Khouang which linked Touby's followers (ultimately Hmong Americans) to Xieng Khouang (Lee M 2015). Given this historical context, the therapeutic landscape in which the Hmong herbal medicines are extracted from provide powerful healing properties as they are grown from the (past) landscapes of Hmong political power.

Consuming Hmong herbal medicine imbues Hmong Americans with the essence of Hmongness that was displaced after America's Secret War. The medicines are socially constructed as "Hmong" and its geographical extraction provide important socio-political contexts in reifying its Hmong essence. The materiality and substantiality of Hmong medicine offer an essential Hmongness that can be readily obtained and imbibed. For Hmong Americans, the trauma of cultural changes, loss of social status, lack of self-worth are all associated with their continual displacement in the United States. The transnational care work network which allows to dispense Hmong medicine seems to offer something solidly Hmong that soothes these sentiments, soothing a larger displacement of Hmong American that explains the importance of its continual practice.

Kaj Siab (Happy): The Hopes of Return

"We all know that they [Hmong Americans with diabetes] are not here for medical treatment because the United States has the best of medicines in the world. They are here to be happy, to be *kaj siab* (peaceful), and to live like they did in their old country." Captured in this fieldwork interview with a Hmong Lao local is the therapeutic landscape of Laos: seeing places of familiarity, reconnecting with displaced family members, courting/marrying Hmong Lao, eating the foods, and enjoying the climate are all material and social embodiments that work to soothe the *nuaj siab* (difficult liver). These returns of Hmong bodies to Laos for healing are caught up with the sentiments of *kaj siab* (to be happy). The mountainous and familial landscapes in Laos work as informal or symbolic sites which are therapeutic in two ways: they contain both the aesthetics of the homeland and the plants used for traditional remedies in the Hmong community. Like Hmong herbal medicines, return to Laos's landscape embodies memory of what it means to be Hmong. In this section, we detail the therapeutic practices of return for Hmong Americans.

In Dr. Thao's work on Hmong American returns, Hmong Americans and their relatives in Laos and Thailand discussed the therapeutics of return as reunification with the old ways of living in Laos and its healing properties serve to return their blood sugar levels to normal. These practices and engagement work together to restore a Hmong American identity. The restoration of a Hmong identity (since chronic disease is caused by displacement) is understood as the healing that interlocutors point to when they state, "In Laos there is a cure for diabetes." As one Hmong Lao living in a village at the outskirts of Vientiane said, "Yes, they come and get to *tham pem* (talk for fun) and we walk and it's like their *mob* (illness) is *kaj siab* (peaceful). Like you're [they're] the old person you [they] left behind and they are better."

Hmong Americans often move through the countries of Laos almost effortlessly. Older Hmong Americans whom Dr. Thao would note as not being able to speak English confidently in the United States were able to order plates of food for themselves and others in Laos. Hmong Americans, in the company of their family members in Laos, traveled the country to see old places of familiarity—the landscape where old villages used to stand—attending Hmong Lao festivities like New Year, and reconnecting with family members.

The arrival of Hmong Americans, and more specifically, the arrival of Hmong American men, often resulted in the elaborate display of familial celebrations. The desire for a temporary and place-specific cure is rooted in the desire to be their old youthful self that had always continued to live in Laos. This, as Dr. Thao understands, is to return to a place where one can be socially mobile, independent, and socially significant as opposed to their life in the United States; this return is ultimately like rejuvenation.

Filial Love (Sib Hlub)

Sib hlub (love) sutures the therapeutic movement of herbs and Hmong American bodies. *Sib hlub* infers that love is reciprocal and, in this case, co-created by Hmong family in the diaspora for healing. Hmong family kinship is delineated by patrilineal and matrilineal lines (*kwvtij neejtsa*). Because family is not delineated by nuclear family, this expansive term of family enables a diasporic network of family. This is especially pertinent in the case of the Hmong diaspora that has been rifted apart from America's War in Laos. Although more women provide the care work in transnational cares, the practices of the family and their engagement with healing Hmong Americans transcend gendered notions of care work.

In this section, we examine the familial relations that support this transnational circulation of medical advices, herbs, and bodies. The Hmong diaspora is known for maintaining very strong relations with their families and communities left behind (Schein 2004, Ogden 2015). "Hmong Americans (. . .) are continuing their relationships with Hmong throughout the world by letters, audiotapes, videotapes, newsletters, e-mail messages, and visits" (Culhane-Pera et al. 2003). Therefore, they maintain a strong sense of cultural identity, and in the medical area they continue to invest in their traditional systems of understanding illness and healing. The consumption of Hmong medicine and the movement of Hmong Americans to Laos is held together by relations in the diaspora, most importantly those that have been torn apart after the war.

Together, medicinal properties of Hmong herbal medicines and Hmong familial relations work to heal the Hmong body. As Hmong herbal medicines are defined as "Hmong," the transnational consumption of Hmong herbal remedies and family participation addresses the symbolic absence of locality and kin. Having family members assist in the search for Hmong medicine, is an act and practice of *sib hlub* and offers soothing qualities to the difficult liver. In Dr. Thao's work, her aunt in Xieng Khouang who is both a shaman and a trained herbalist, said "Selling Hmong medicine is all a business" as they crouched down to examine the herbs of an elderly Hmong Lao woman who brought the herbs to Phonsavan all the way from Nong Het, a 3-hour two rail truck ride away. Dr. Thao observed that the woman selling the herbs, a *niam tais* (grandmother) who had on gold earrings and gold rings, a display of wealth. "You have to know what's good and what's not, and sometimes it's just a tree." In other words, sometimes the herbs sold as medicine are not at all medicinal. The pursuit of Hmong medicine must be vetted through the family who plays the central role of care worker. Unlike in the U.S. where Hmong American patients see the doctor individually and are then treated, seeking Hmong medicine in Laos and Thailand is a social endeavor that brings together family in hopes of healing the sick. It is an act of love.

The transnational circulation of care also includes the transfer of advice through telephone calls and internet. A man was about to send a parcel to his brother-in-law when we met him at the Post Office in a village called "km52" (i.e., 52 kilometers from the capital Vientiane). "This is the first time I send plants to Fresno (California), however, I regularly send traditional clothes and embroidery. My brother-in-law called me several times because he has a stomach ache; he described his symptoms and asked me to send him treatment (a farmer in km52 village, Laos)." During the interview, he explained how he learned to cure with plants by his mother and repeated several times that he did not understand why his brother-in-law in the United States needed these plants for treatment. After several phone calls, he finally went to collect the plants himself in the province of Xieng Khouang. This example emphasizes that, from the point of view of the Hmong who remain in Laos, it is not necessarily easy to understand why the Hmong abroad ask for medical advice from their relatives and still use herbal medicine from Laos while they have access to a modern health care system and well trained doctors. Nevertheless, the transnational healing process tends to strengthen the unity of the family and serves as a reminder of the importance of close family ties and by extension the community solidarity.

Hmong Americans use their transnational linkages to find the right treatment for their sickness. In Dr. Bochaton's work, parcel shipments and the medicinal flows tend to fill the gaps of the U.S. health system. Although some plants are ideally used fresh in Laos, the plants sent abroad are dried before being prepared for transportation in plastic bags. In addition to these large scale medicinal movements from Laos to the United States, the transnational circulation of care also happens in suitcases through personal travel of Hmong Americans on their way back to their host country. Several plant sellers met in km52 and Phonsavan markets reported that Hmong American sometimes buy plants in Laos and bring them to the United States; these purchases are usually made in December at the time of Hmong New Year which attracts many Hmong living in the U.S.

Family in the U.S. also supports the circulation of herbal healers who travel from Laos. Sponsored by family in the U.S. they bring with them luggage full of freshly harvested and dried medicinal plants. "I went twice to the U.S. in 2006 and 2007 to visit but also to sell medicinal plants (about 60 kg of goods each time). Three of my daughters live in Oklahoma and Michigan. I went to the U.S. with my husband and I sold to relatives and acquaintances there" (healer in Nong Het district). This healer met in Nong Het brought with her a document prepared by Phonsavan hospital allowing her to leave Laos with the plants and take them through the U.S. customs. She explained she earned about US$3,000 each time.

Hmong Americans who return to Laos seek out family members who are knowledgeable about herbs. They are often requested to gather large bags of herbs for their relatives with chronic diseases like diabetes. Family members along with herbal healers boil the herbs in a cauldron in such a quantity that the atmosphere seems like an herbal sauna. The afflicted person sits in the middle and bathes in the herbs. Its medicinal properties are absorbed into the body. These are "the everyday techniques through which individuals, even if they are of modest means, comfort themselves, compensate for daily difficulties and frustrations, or build a life of reliable bodily satisfactions" (Farquhar, 1994:481). In the company of family and in the social networks of family, these are the practices that make healing possible.

Returning home appears as an alternative practice of care within a classic therapeutic itinerary. As mentioned earlier, it echoes the notion of "therapeutic landscapes" developed by Gesler (1992) and briefly defined as "places that have achieved lasting reputations for providing physical, mental and spiritual healing" (Kearns and Gesler 1998, 8). These returns involve a strong element of hope and touch upon questions of cultural identity among the Hmong diaspora. The emphasis on family and familial love challenges gendered notions of care work, illustrating the ways family in Laos, where both men and women participate in caring for Hmong American ailments. Nevertheless as Baldassar & Merla show in their book (2014) "transnational caregiving [. . .] binds members together in intergenerational networks of reciprocity and obligation, love and trust, that are simultaneously fraught with tension, contest, and relations of unequal power" (p. 7).

Ambivalence: Frictions, Capital, and Power

Hmong transnational cares creates an economy of reciprocity between Hmong American and Hmong Laos. Through the material practices of finding and consuming herbs to the practices of receiving Hmong Americans in Laos, the exchange of care work restructures and reinforces the ties between the two that was displaced because of America's War in Laos. The economy of reciprocity and Hmong Lao discourses of reception around the Hmong American creates a homogenous community despite historical divergences and contradictions, moving beyond patriarchal, gendered, and ethno-national formations of Hmong. At the same time, this homogenous community is caught within the frictions of globalization and the inequalities produced from U.S. imperialism and French colonialism in Laos. In this section, we detail the social, historical, and economic ambivalences embedded within this therapeutic landscape.

Sentiments of nostalgia and loss are deeply embedded in the Hmong diaspora. Hmong Lao address these sentiments when they call the Hmong American "home" Using the words *los* and *tuaj* means "to come" in English. But the differentiation between the words *los* and *tuaj* is the interpellation of a subject as kin (patrilineal) or as outsider (matrilineal/others). In Hmong, the word *los* designates that the individual has returned to a place of *home* or a place of family, whereas the word *tuaj* means the person is visiting. Family and home are conflated within the word *los*. In Dr. Thao's (2018a) observations and argument, "*koj los*" was used for all Hmong Americans irrespective of whether the person hailing them was of kin (*kwvtij*), queering Hmong patriarchal practices. It is in this ambiguity, this departure from Hmong patriarchal practices of interpellation, that a homogenous Hmong community in diaspora is created.

Creating Hmong Americans and Hmong Lao as occupying a homogenous community, Hmong Lao also describe themselves as those who were left behind by their Hmong American family members. This discourse conscripts Hmong Americans as not refugees who fled Laos during Pathet Lao reappraisal toward American sympathizers in the country but rather sees Hmong Americans as migrants who chose to leave Hmong Lao. This narration erases the historical specificity of the multiple motivations for Hmong Lao who stayed in Laos. Some didn't align themselves with the Americans but rather the Pathet Lao party. Some retreated into the dense forests of Xieng Khouang and fought as resistance fighters until surrender and were afterwards relocated by the Lao government into various areas such as Vientiane. These types of discourse work to remap Hmong Americans as always belonging in Laos despite the historical trauma of the war in Laos and even current day tensions and hostilities between Hmong American and Hmong Lao. Hmong patriarchal practices and ethno-national narratives of community are revised for the creation of a homogenous Hmong community.

Creating a homogenous Hmong community in diaspora makes possible the commodification of transnational care. In Dr. Thao's ethnography, she notices that those with family in the United States are often wealthier. Hmong Lao young women are often encouraged to marry older and sometimes elderly Hmong American men as a prospect for building wealth. The reverse is also encouraged, where young Hmong Lao men also marry elderly Hmong American women as well, however, that union is often more stigmatized. Marriage socially and culturally cements Hmong American and Hmong Lao relationships into kinship. Hmong American returns for healing sometimes resulted in transnational marriages. In Dr. Bochaton's work, the economy of herbal plants has also provided many opportunities of economic wealth for Hmong Lao. The increase in sales of plants to the United States has gradually required new recruits to increase their supplies of plants. Vendors from km52 village gradually involved their daughters, sisters, cousins, nieces in the business by asking them to send plants regularly by bus (the bags of plants are placed in the bunkers and the journey takes about 10–12 hours), once a month during the rainy season and two or three times per month during the dry season on average. The volumes of plants collected and delivered range from 10 kg up to 80 kg each time. Hmong pickers (who are mainly from the same clan) decided in turn to sell on Tam Say (Nong Het District Center) market every Saturday morning in order to gain new customers and increase plant purchases. Due to a snowball effect, women living in remote villages (2–3 hours walk from Tam Say) are also involved in this business as plant gatherers.

The incomes of women involved in the medicinal plants trade depend on the role they play in the sector: pickers, intermediaries, sellers, healers. It also depends on how closely and directly they are connected to the transnational market. The pickers from Nong Het district are the first link in the supply chain and earn a moderate income: from US$100/year for the least regular pickers to US$400/year for the pickers who have contacts with numerous customers and collect plants regularly. Among gatherers encountered in Tam Say market, one stated: *"it's a good business because customers sometimes order 100 or 200 kg of plants. That's a lot of money."* According to the women interviewed, these additional incomes mostly allow them to send children to school and to buy food.

The pickers with relatives established in the United States enjoy higher incomes as they have the opportunity to send plants without hiring the services of intermediaries. A woman whose sister left Laos to settle in the U.S. very recently, already received five orders of medicinal plants (between 5 and 8 kg). Her sister calls her and describes the type and the amount of plants she needs. After picking, she sends the raw herbs and once they reach the U.S., they are cut into pieces and packaged. Her sister often makes mixtures of several plants to treat high blood pressure, gastric problems (stomach burn), and overweight. "My sister seems to earn a good living there. When I send her some plants, she often sends me back 200-300 US$." The opportunity of direct transactions with the U.S. is highly pursued: a woman from km52 wanted to send some plants to her relatives living in the U.S. so that they could sell on-site. "But my cousins are very busy, they do not have time to do that. So I've never sent anything at the moment" (saleswoman in km52). Two women from Nong Het district who started this business at an early stage are now the main negotiators between pickers and resellers in the markets in Laos and abroad. The income they derive from this full-time activity approximates US$ 300–400/month which brings them a very comfortable income supplement in addition to the cultivation of rice. The herb vendors in the markets have the highest incomes but these vary with the seasons. A woman from km52 stated she earned between US$40 and US$120/day. Her Hmong customers come from the surrounding villages and even from Thailand, France, and the United States.

Despite the contradictions and ambivalences in constructing Hmong herbs and Hmong American returns to Laos as possible practices of engagement for healing, this section shows the ways these therapeutic mobilities work to create a homogenous community that transcends normative practices of Hmong patriarchy, gender, and ethno-national formations. Reception of Hmong Americans in Laos and the engagement of Hmong Lao family members for healing structures an economy of reciprocity that binds Hmong Americans to Hmong Laos either through marriage or the creation of a transnational market. It also offers up economic possibilities for Hmong Lao, and specifically for Hmong Lao women who are able to generate income. This case study demonstrates the accuracy of the "love and money framework" to conceptualize the notion of care work as it argues "against dichotomous views in which markets are seen as antithetical to true care, and against the view that true care can only be found in families" (England 2005).

CONCLUSION

Medicine, and particularly medicine as developed in the West (biomedicine), for older Hmong Americans is deeply racialized and cultural. Hmong past experiences in Laos to resettlement and encounters with biomedicine, illustrate that medicine is situated within the intersections of imperialism, religious conversions, and racial discrimination. Hmong Americans' engagement within a transnational circulation of care (between Laos and the U.S.) critiques biomedicine's colonial and imperial past and seeks a form of healing for Hmong American displacement in the U.S. Through the practices and enactments of familial love and consumption of Hmong "traditional" healing, this transnational circulation of care forms a strong social field in the Hmong diaspora.

Hmong herbs and returns to Laos for health and healing are appealing and are seen to contain a "power of healing in themselves" (van der Geest and Whyte, 1989:346), because in their consumption and the act of return, these forms of care help to treat the ills of displacement that is embodied and materialized as chronic disease symptoms. The hopes of healing the difficult/ distressed liver encompass multiple practices and pleasures of healing: the materiality of Hmong herbs, where Hmong herbs are cultivated from, the familial practices surrounding the sale and consumption of Hmong herbal medicines. In addition, what makes the herbs and return appealing are also the actors of Hmong Lao and the therapeutic landscapes of Laos. Hmong Lao care work, the exchanges of familial love and hope, and the affective components of Laos's landscape soothes the Hmong American difficult liver (*nyuaj siab*) and the source of that difficult liver, the displacement of Hmong Americans, their kinship, and Hmong identity.

Far from Western assumptions that healthcare is just a private concern of family members, these transnational care exchanges within the Hmong diaspora are embedded in the broader political, economic, cultural, and social context of both sending and receiving societies. Affects of hope, love, and ambivalence are at the crossroad of this commoditized transnational quest for care. Hmong familial love and hope structures a homogenous Hmong community, revising the historical conflicts and tensions of Hmong American relationships to Hmong Lao. By queering care work, transgressing Hmong patriarchal practices and ethno-national narratives of community, we also argue that queering care work facilitates healing a displaced Hmong body politic. Perhaps, it also infers their indebtedness to one another for healing and survival in the aftermath of Western imperialism.

The mountainous landscapes of Laos act as informal or symbolic sites which are therapeutic and work as a memory of what it means to be Hmong. Paradoxically, the desire to embody the aesthetics of Hmong original landscape (Odgen 2015), consumption of Hmong herbal medicines in the Hmong diaspora, and its global commodification may disrupt this therapeutic landscape. We are aware that this notion of a Hmong original landscape is itself a form of romanticization, as if Laos has remained untouched after Hmong American exodus from Laos. Further examination needs to situate Laos' relationship to the global economy and the exports of Laos' natural resources (including Hmong herbal medicines). An issue not examined in this chapter is the impact of transnational circulation of herbs on the local ecosystem from which they originate. This concerns the pressure asserted onto Hmong Lao to pick more herbal plants from the forests of Northern Laos for export (Bochaton 2018). There needs to be further examination of these herbal plant collections, who else are consumers of these herbs, to which countries are they sent to, and its impact on the ecology. With increasing globalization of Laos and this commoditized care, we wonder what form Hmong transnational circulation of care will take within the Hmong diaspora amid climate change and ongoing globalization.

NOTES

1. The Hmong diaspora is more expansive than just Laos and the United States. The Hmong diaspora spans the United States, France, French Guiana, German, and Australia. While we recognize that there are mobilities from these countries to Laos, there remains a unique pattern between Laos and the United States that structures the majority of mobilities to Laos to be specifically from the United States. This is most likely representative of the United States's involvement in recruiting Hmong in Laos as proxy fighters during the Vietnam War. Therefore, when we speak about the mobility between Hmong in the United States and Laos, we use the term transnationalism defined as "immigrants build social fields that link together their country of origin and their country of settlement" (Glick Schiller, Basch, Blanc-Szanton 1992, 1).

2. This idea of queering the Hmong diaspora was a conversation between author Mai See Thao and colleague Kong Pheng Pha. We draw on Pha's dissertation (2017) to inform our understanding of how Hmong transnational cares queer care work. He writes, "The conditions of the past enable queer materializations of community, but in that process, changes and produces heterogeneities that controverts the promise of a universal communal liberation." (p. 266)

3. In Langford's (2013) book Consoling Ghosts: Stories of Medicine and Mourning from Southeast Asians in Exile, she describes a Hmong economy of barter between the living and the dead. Citing the late anthropologist Nicholas Tapp (1989), Langford writes, that the connection between the living and the dead is bridged together through a marketplace where the communities "trade, deal, and bargain with each other" (Tapp, 1989, 64).These kinds of exchanges differ from transactionable goods, these exchanges insist on a relationship between the two communities. Using the notion of the gift, Langford compellingly argues that these exchanges are "rooted less in utilitarian obligation than in persistent connection and love. However, once again, an expressivisit witnessing is not what the dead primarily ask of that love. . . . They ask instead that it be manifest in physical gifts and actions. They require companionship, hospitality, a good view from their burial sites. This materiality signals not a narrowly interested exchange, but a continuous current of care flown in several directions at once, defying the spilt between autology and genealogy" (180–181). We find this similar kind of reciprocity and exchange shape and structure the transnational cares specifically in returns to Laos for care/cure. In our manuscript what is demonstrated is the tension between two economies, one of commodities and one of reciprocity.

4. Depression often denotes an individualized experience that is thought to be an interior experience, whether that is by chemical changes in the brain or to one's own personal traumas that is internalized. *Kev nyuaj siab* in the Hmong translation resists an internalization of depression and insists on the attention to the social context. See Thao MS 2018 dissertation.

BIBLIOGRAPHY

Baldassar L., Merla L. (eds.), 2014. *Transnational Families, Migration and the Circulation of Care. Understanding Mobility and Absence in Family Life.* New York, London: Routledge, p. 320.

Bochaton, A. 2018. "Intertwined Therapeutic Mobilities: Knowledge, Plants, Healers on the Move between Laos and the U.S." *Mobilities*, DOI: 10.1080/17450101.2018.1522878

Chan, S. 1991. *Asian Americans : An Interpretive History.* Boston: Twayne Publishers.

Chan, S. 1994. *Hmong Means Free: Life in Laos and America.* Philadelphia: Temple University Press.

Chiu, M. 2004. "Medical, Racist, and Colonial Constructions of Power: Creating the Asian American Patient and the Cultural Citizen in Anne Fadiman's The Spirit Catches You and You Fall Down." *Hmong Studies Journal* 5: 1–36.

Corlett, J. L., E. A. Dean, and L. E. Grivetti. 2003. "Hmong Gardens: Botanical Diversity in an Urban Setting." *Economic Botany* 57 (3): 365–379. doi:10.1663/0013-0001.

Culhane-Pera, K. A., D. E. Vawter, P. Xiong, B. Babbitt, and M. M. Solberg. 2003. *Healing by Heart: Clinical and Ethical Case Stories of Hmong Families and Western Providers.* Nashville: Vanderbilt University Press.

Culhane-Pera, K. A., Cheng Her, and Bee Her. 2007. "'We Are out of Balance Here': A Hmong Cultural Model of Diabetes." *Journal of Immigrant and Minority Health* 9 (3): 179–90. DOI: 10.1007/s10903-006-9029-3.

Dia, C. 2003. *Hmong American Concepts of Health.* New York and London: Routledge.

Dilger, H., A. Kane, and S. Langwick. 2012. *Medicine, Mobility, and Power in Global Africa: Transnational Health and Healing.* Bloomington: Indiana University Press.

England, P. 2005. "Emerging Theories of Care Work." *Annual Review of Sociology* 31: 381–399.

Fadiman, A. 1998. *The Spirit Catches You and You Fall Down: A Hmong Child, Her American Doctors, and the Collision of Two Cultures.* New York: Farrar: Strauss and Giroux.

Farquhar, J. 1994. "Eating Chinese Medicine." *Cultural Anthropology* 9 (4): 471–97.

Geest, Sjaak Van Der, and Susan Reynolds Whyte. 1989. "The Charm of Medicines: Metaphors and Metonyms." *Medical Anthropology Quarterly, New Series* 3 (4): 345–67.

Gesler, W. 1992. "Therapeutic Landscapes: Medical Issues in Light of the New Cultural Geography." *Social Science and Medicine* 3: 735–746. doi:10.1016/0277-9536(92)90360-3.

Glick Schiller, Nina, Linda Basch, and Cristina Blanc-Szanton. 1992. "Transnationalism: A New Analytic Framework for Understanding Migration." *Annals of New York Academy of Sciences* 645 (1): 1–24.

Hamilton-Merritt, J. 1993. *Tragic Mountains : The Hmong, the Americans, and the Secret Wars for Laos, 1942–1992.* Bloomington: Indiana University Press.

Henry, R. R. 1996. "Sweet Blood, Dry Liver: Diabetes and Hmong Embodiment in a Foreign Land." University of North Carolina at Chapel Hill.

Hillmer, Paul. 2010. *A People's History of the Hmong*. St. Paul: Minnesota Historical Society Press.

Hondagneu-Sotelo, P. 2001. *Domestica: Immigrant Workers Cleaning and Caring in the Shadows of Affluence*. Berkeley: University of California Press.

Hochschild, A.R. 2000. "The Nanny Chain." *American Prospect* 11:32–36.

Kane, A. 2012. "Flows of Medicine, Healers, Health Professionals, and Patients between Home and Host Countries." In *Medicine, Mobility and Power in Global Africa: Transnational Health and Healing*, edited by H. Dilger, A. Kane, and S. Langwick, 190–212. Bloomington: Indiana University Press.

Kangas, B., 2007 "Hope from Abroad in the International Medical Travel of Yemeni Patients" *Anthropology & Medicine* 14(3): 293–305. DOI: 10.1080/13648470701612646

Kearns, R. A., and W. M. Gesler. 1998. "Introduction." In *Putting Health into Place: Landscape, Identity and Well-Being*, edited by A. Robin, R. Kearns, and W. M. Gesler, 1–16. Syracuse, NY: Syracuse University Press.

Langford, J. 2013. *Consoling Ghosts : Stories of Medicine and Mourning from Southeast Asians in Exile*. Minneapolis: University of Minnesota Press.

Lee, G. Y., 1982. "Minority Policies and the Hmong in Laos." In *Contemporary Laos: Studies in the Politics and Society of the Lao People's Democratic Republic*, edited by Stuart-Fox, M.. New York: St Martin Press.

Lee, M. N. M. 2015. *Dreams of the Hmong Kingdom : The Quest for Legitimation in French Indochina, 1850–1960*. Madison: The University of Wisconsin Press.

Lee, M. N. M. 2018. "The Origin and Creation of Hmong American Memories of Blood Sacrifice of the United States During the Secret War." Oral Presentation. Hmong Studies Consortium. Madison, WI. 5/3/2018.

Mignot, F. 2003. *Santé et Intégration Nationale au Laos: Rencontres Entre Montagnards et Gens des Plaines*. Paris: L'Harmattan.

Ogden, M. 2015. "Tebchaws: A Theory of Magnetic Media and Hmong Diasporic Homeland." *Hmong Studies Journal* 16: 1–25.

Perriam, G. 2015. Sacred Spaces, Healing Places: Therapeutic Landscapes of Spiritual Significance. *Journal of Medical Humanities* 36 (1):19–33.

Pha, K. P. 2017. "Queer Refugeeism: Constructions of Race, Gender, and Sexuality in the Hmong Diaspora." University of Minnesota-Twin Cities.

Schein, L. 2004. "Homeland Beauty: Transnational Longing and Hmong American Video." *The Journal of Asian Studies* 63 (2): 433–63. https://doi.org/10.1017/S0021911804001032.

Stuart-Fox, M. 1997. *A History of Laos*. Cambridge, U.K.; New York, NY: Cambridge University Press.

Taylor, J. S. 2003a. "Confronting '"Culture"' in Medicine's '"Culture of No Culture.'"" *Academic Medicine* 78 (6): 555–59. papers3://publication/uuid/306 2D745-16FD-492A-8630-A59FDA3B1763.

Taylor, J. S. 2003b. "The Story Catches You and You Fall Down: Tragedy, Ethnography, and 'Cultural Competence'." *Medical Anthropology Quarterly* 17 (2): 159–81. https://doi.org/10.1525/maq.2003.17.2.159.

Thao, MS. 2018a. "Bittersweet Migrations: Type II Diabetes and Healing in the Hmong Diaspora." University of Minnesota-Twin Cities.

Thao, MS. 2018b. "The Politics of Culture in Medicine." Invited Lecture. Asian Pacific American Medical Student Association Lunch Series. Medical College of Wisconsin. Milwaukee, WI.

Thao, MS. 2019. "Kev Nyuaj Siab (The Distressed/Difficult Liver): Tracing Displacement and Loss in Type II Diabetes for Older Hmong Americans."

Tiilikainen, M. 2012. "It's Just like the Internet: Transnational Healing Practices between Somaliland and the Somali Diaspora." In *Medicine, Mobility and Power in Global Africa: Transnational Health and Healing*, edited by H. Dilger, A. Kane, and S. Langwick, 271–294. Bloomington: Indiana University Press.

Tsing, A. L. 2005. *Friction: An Ethnography of Global Connection*. Princeton: Princeton University Press.

Vang, M. 2012. "Displaced Histories: Refugee Critique and the Politics of Hmong American Remembering." University of California San Diego. https://doi.org/10.1300/J122v22n03_06.

Vang, C. Y. 2010. *Hmong America : Reconstructing Community in Diaspora*. Urbana: University of Illinois Press.

Weldon, C. 1999. *Tragedy in Paradise: A Country Doctor at War in Laos*. Bangkok: Asia Books.

Williams, A. 1998. "Therapeutic Landscapes in Holistic Medicine." *Social Sciences and Medicine* 46(9): 1193–1203.

Williams, A. (Ed.), 2007. *Therapeutic Landscapes*. Hampshire, UK: Ashgate Publishing Limited, p. 400.

Wright, A. 1986. "A Never Ending Refugee Camp: The Explosive Birthrate in Ban Vinai." Unpublished paper. Bangkok, Thailand.

Yun M. 2010. *Commercializing Hmong Used Clothing: The Transnational Trade in Hmong Textiles Across the Mekong Region*, The Regional Center for Social Science and Sustainable Development (RCSD) Faculty of Social Sciences, Chiang Mai University, 19p.

Chapter 2

Informal Caregiving in a Transnational Context

The Case of Canadian International Retirement Migrants in the United States

Valorie A. Crooks and John Pickering

Worldwide, and especially among those living within the Global North, growing numbers of older people are opting to participate in international retirement migration. Sometimes referred to as amenity migration or sunshine migration (Hass 2013), short-term international migration occurs when older people move across national borders to spend weeks or months of the year in another country (Pickering and Crooks 2019). Our own recent scoping review of the international literature has found that people choose to participate in this mobility based primarily on four main factors, which are those related to (1) the destination (e.g., climate), (2) people (e.g., potential for creating friendships and socializing), (3) cost (e.g., housing affordability), and (4) movement (e.g., ease of travel) (ibid). In addition to being interested in living abroad, older persons who are considering international migration as a viable option need to have the financial capital required to spend significant lengths of time in another country (Sunil et al. 2007) and the social skills and cultural capital that will enable them to integrate into a new environment (Coates et al 2002; Longino et al. 2002). Health and wellbeing are also important enablers to participation, in that international retirement migrants must have the physical and mental ability to travel and live abroad and also access to resources (e.g., travel health insurance, health care clinics, medical records) to manage any health exacerbations while away (Pickering et al. 2019). For those coping with complex chronic conditions, multiple diagnoses, significant mobility impairments, and/or limited mental capacity, traveling abroad with someone else who can assist with providing informal care—such as a spouse, partner, friend, or family member—is likely another important enabler to participating in international retirement migration.

Many thousands of older Canadians participate in international retirement migration each year. They are often looking to spend weeks or months in warmer destinations with favorable climates while avoiding winter, and the limited mobility that it can bring about, at home. While there is no formal tracking and tracing of these transnational movements, it is estimated that somewhere between 500,000 to more than one million older Canadians travel to destinations in the United States alone each year to stay for an extended period of time during winter (Coates et al. 2002; Desrosiers-Lauzon 2009). Other popular destinations for these Canadian retirement migrants include locations in Mexico and countries in Central America and the Caribbean. As Canadian international retirement migrants are typically in their sixties or beyond, it is common for travelers to be managing one or more chronic health conditions, to be in some form of recovery from an acute health episode, and/or to experience a health exacerbation or event while abroad (Coates et al. 2002). This may necessitate some to access formal health care while abroad (Marshall et al. 1989). Our own recent research in the popular U.S. destination of Yuma, Arizona has found that the presence of Canadian international retirement migrants in need of medical care can present both opportunities and challenges for local hospitals and health care workers (ibid). Challenges can include facilitating continuity of care in this transnational context and the lack of familiarity with patients' home health care systems, while opportunities can allow for increased staffing at facilities and the creation of novel community-based outreach programs. Certainly, much care for Canadian snowbirds who are managing chronic or acute health conditions actually happens outside the hospital and is informal in nature. This is because most care work among Canadians is performed by informal caregivers, often unpaid and untrained friends and family members, who provide a range of physical, social, emotional, and financial care to those managing chronic, acute, and/or long-term health conditions (Romanow 2002).

Informal caregivers play an important role in health management. The quality and availability of informal care someone is able to access is directly related to their own health status as a care recipient, and thus such care shapes health status and health outcomes (Nijboer et al. 2001). When informal caregivers have access to the supports they need to assist them with their care duties—whether practical, financial, social, emotional, or otherwise—the health of care recipients is strengthened (Mittelman et al. 2006). Meanwhile, when informal caregivers lack access to needed personal, medical, and financial supports this may bring about stress and anxiety that can lead to the onset of caregiver burden (Carretero et al. 2009; Sisk 2000). Thus, the health and wellbeing of informal caregivers in any context, who are typically family members of friends of the care recipient, can be compromised or negatively impacted through the practice of providing care. Oppositely, supporting family members and friends to care for those managing chronic and acute health conditions by providing meaningful resources, including informational interventions, can assist with lessening the likelihood of the onset of caregiver burden (Fast and Keating 2000). Existing research has shown that such resources need to consider the specific context or environment in which care happens as different care settings can bring up different support needs for informal caregivers (Callan 2007; Giesbrecht et al. 2010; Stajduhar 2003).

International retirement migration is a particular care context for informal caregivers given that it is a transnational practice and thus the friends and family who provide care are likely doing so both at home and abroad—our previous research on the transnational practice of medical tourism has documented this to be the case in that care context (Crooks et al. 2017; Whitmore et al. 2019). These caregivers and those they care for cross national borders, the focus of which in this chapter involves traveling from Canada to the United States, and thus they actually temporarily move away from the health systems and the support systems that actually enable care and health management on an ongoing basis. However, very little is actually known about how informal caregiving occurs in the international retirement migration context. In this chapter, we address this particular knowledge gap through reporting on what we learned from dyad interviews (n = 10 interviews, 20 participants) conducted with Canadian informal caregivers and the partners they care for while abroad for the winter. These dyad interviews were conducted in-person with Canadians wintering in Yuma, Arizona in over a two-week period in January of 2019. Yuma is a warm, dry city in southern Arizona that borders with Mexico and has a year-round population of almost 100,000 that typically doubles in the winter with Canadian and American retirement migrants. We recruited people to participate in interviews through social media advertising and by placing informational post cards containing study information on the driver-side windows of vehicles with Canadian license plates. While we were open to all types of caregiving dyads (e.g., friends who travel together, siblings, or other family members), all participants were heterosexual marital partners where one partner had defined care needs as a result of chronic or acute illness. In the coming sections, we present five unique vignettes based on a narrative review of the interviews that highlight specific dimensions of the practice of informal caregiving in the context of international retirement migration among Canadian marital partners. While these vignettes are drawn from participants' lived experiences, pseudonyms are used and all identifying information has been removed to maintain anonymity.

VIGNETTE 1: DINA AND PAUL

Dina and Paul lived in the Canadian province of Ontario and had spent the last five winters in Yuma in a rented trailer. Dina had an ongoing chronic condition that had a serious exacerbation requiring extensive medical intervention, and ultimately surgery, during a previous trip to Yuma. She was hospitalized in Yuma for several days to stabilize her symptoms, after which it was determined that she required surgery. While the physicians treating her in Yuma wanted Dina to have surgery there, her travel health insurance provider required her to return home to Canada for care. This was not unexpected given that Canadians typically purchase *travel* health insurance policies to cover them while in the United States, which may result in an insurer covering the cost of returning home for care if one's health is stable enough instead of receiving treatment abroad, as opposed to comprehensive medical insurance (Marshall et al. 1989). Dina and Paul both found it stressful to follow the decision-making around where the surgery would be performed, whether in Yuma or upon quick return to Canada, as the information they could access was limited and was also sometimes contradictory. Paul attempted to clarify these details as often as he could in addition to maintaining a steady channel of communication with the travel health insurance provider. As Dina explained, "And most of it [waiting for surgery] is trying to find out, okay, what's going to happen? What are they going to do? When is it going to happen? Where's it going to happen? And as it gets dragged out, you know, you start to get a little more anxious." Ultimately Dina was flown back to Canada, where she was immediately taken into hospital to be stabilized and prepared for surgery, while Paul drove back to meet her there. Their separation was necessary as Paul needed to pack up their belongings in Yuma, clean their rented accommodations, and return to Canada with their vehicle.

While Paul routinely assisted Dina with managing her health both at home and while in the United States, when her symptoms exacerbated to the point of requiring hospitalization in Yuma, he had to take on significant caregiving responsibilities. These responsibilities reflected their transnational care context in that he had to liaise with the travel health insurance provider they had purchased a policy from about care options in the United States and Canada, navigate packing up quickly in Yuma for an unexpected early end to their time there, and assisting Dina with re-entry into the health care system at home upon her return there. His care responsibilities centered heavily on gathering and communicating information about Dina's health and specific medical tests to physicians, along with keeping friends and family updated both in Yuma and at home. This role had a great deal of complexity because upon return to Canada and admission to hospital there, Dina's physicians requested copies of her medical records. Paul provided the records, only to learn that "there's a difference between the [medical record] systems here [in Yuma], and the systems up in Canada when it comes to reading tests . . . I don't know what it was, because they sent us with all the reports, and everything [but they weren't reported in the ways the doctors wanted to see them." Paul also had to spend a significant amount of time relaying information, both health and details of travel logistics, to their travel health policy insurer.

Paul's experience of providing informal care to Dina in the context of international retirement migrants signals an important dimension of this transnational caregiving experience, which is that caregivers are often expected to share, retain, and remember important health information to assist with coordinating care (Weinberg et al. 2007). In effect, they are playing a role in facilitating transnational informational continuity of care for the care recipient. Establishing a continuous medical record, having a regular care provider, and coordinating care transitions are hallmarks of care continuity (Cho et al. 2015; Crooks and Agarwal 2008; Haggerty et al. 2003), and when someone needs to access care while away from home it is difficult-to-impossible to have such continuity. Meanwhile, experiencing continuity of care is associated with better health and health outcomes, especially for those managing chronic conditions (Manious et al. 2004). Away from their home health system and usual health care providers, Paul stepped in to assist with facilitating informational continuity of care for Dina by gathering information from multiple sources (e.g., travel health insurer, physicians in Yuma, surgeons in Ontario). A study that explored informal caregiving in medical tourism, which is a transnational practice that involves travel abroad with the intent of accessing medical care, indicated that facilitating information transfer (or informational continuity) is part of a larger knowledge broker role that informal caregivers take on when they are caring for someone who is accessing care abroad (Casey et al. 2013). Other aspects of the knowledge broker role taken on by informal caregivers providing care in a transnational context include asking questions on behalf of care recipients, clearly relaying information to care recipients, translating information as needed, and retaining information. Other than translating information into another language, Paul's experience of caring for Dina and facilitating continuity in the process of doing so reflects the key aspects of this knowledge broker role.

VIGNETTE 2: FRANCINE AND FRANK

Francine and Frank lived in Western Canada and had traveled seasonally to Yuma, Arizona for the past many years. They would drive to Yuma in a motorhome and live in it while abroad. Francine was the main caregiver and prior to traveling to Yuma she would fill prescriptions and make copies of recent medical records so they could have those items on-hand in the motorhome in the chance they were needed. Their goal was to take with them all the supplies they will need to manage their health while in Yuma so that they could avoid costly out-of-pocket health care payments while in the United States. As Francine explained, "We sort of have to cover all the things that might happen and bring it [prescriptions, over-the-counter medications], so and then find a space for it [in the motorhome])." They believed that spending time in the warm, dry climate of Southern Arizona was also health promoting and that this lessened the likelihood of negative health events while living away from home.

During a previous summer in Yuma, Frank experienced an exacerbation of a pre-existing dental problem and required immediate attention. They opted to drive south of Yuma to Los Algodones, Mexico where Frank was able to access dental care quickly and affordably. They returned to Yuma, where Frank recuperated and Francine cared for him. She prepared soft foods, including soups, and monitored his overall health. In another instance, Frank had to visit an urgent care center in Yuma when he injured his finger. Once again, Francine monitored his pain levels and medications as he recovered from this injury. Frank did not have any significant ongoing chronic health conditions, and thus Francine's experience of providing care while in Yuma was defined by these two relatively minor acute care situations. In fact, she did not consider herself to be an informal caregiver and viewed her care work to be "just regular married stuff."

Francine was not alone in her belief that informal care work is nothing special and simply part of her marital relationship. In fact, this sentiment was echoed by many of those who participated in these dyad interviews. Much research has established the invisibility of the care work performed by friends and family members, especially because it occurs in the private space of the home, and this invisibility is compounded when caregivers do not view themselves as such nor consider their responsibilities to be care work (Dahlborg Lyckhage and Lindahl 2013; Herd and Meyer 2002; Villalobos Dintrans 2019). The invisibility of care work combined with the fact that many consider it to be a normal part of family and friend relationships can pose a number of risks. A significant risk is that such care work can become undervalued, which many argue that it is and has been so for decades in both medical and social spheres (Carmichael and Ercolani 2014; Murphey et al. 2007). Another risk is that the invisibility and undervaluing of informal care work and thus informal caregivers results in them not being considered as members of the care team by health care professionals and thus not consulted during decision-making (Gillick 2013; Shen et al. 2020). Finally, those who consider care work to be "just regular married stuff" and do not identify as caregivers may miss out on resources that are targeted to support their own health and the care they provide, such as support groups and informational tools. This has particular implications for caregiver support in the context of international retirement migration as caregivers are removed from the social and family support networks they have curated at home and thus may experience particular losses through not identifying as informal caregivers while abroad. Meanwhile, it has been established that older caregivers, such as those who are post-retirement (e.g., international retirement migrants), provide more intensive care work and a greater number of care hours than younger caregivers and are thus in most need of having support (Carmichael and Ercolani 2014).

VIGNETTE 3: GERTRUDE AND PRESTON

Gertrude and Preston were married partners who lived in the Canadian province of British Columbia. For the previous five winters they had made Yuma, Arizona their home-away-from-home as international retirement migrants. They were both in their early seventies and considered themselves to be in good health. Preston had a history of heart disease and had prior heart surgeries and took medication to manage his symptoms. In a previous winter visit to Yuma, however, Preston had a significant, acute heart health event that required major medical intervention despite his cardiologist at home considering his condition stable and approving him for travel. Gertrude called their travel health insurance policy provider when Preston's symptoms intensified, and they instructed her to take him to the local hospital's urgent care center in Yuma. His symptoms were assessed, he was stabilized and prescribed medications, and then was sent home. The next day he became disoriented and was unable to communicate properly. Gertrude had a friend from their retirement trailer park take them to the hospital, where Preston was treated and discharged again. The next day the hospital called to explain that he needed to be admitted for intensive care immediately and asked that Gertrude bring all of Preston's medical records with him. Fortunately, she had brought copies with her from Canada, which was typical of the care work she performed to assist Preston with managing his heart health. Preston remained in the hospital in Yuma for many days, the costs of which were covered by his travel health insurance provider (not without some extensive negotiation, though), and once he was stable enough to do so he returned to Canada for bypass surgery.

Gertrude was thrust into a heightened caregiving role while abroad in Yuma that involved responsibilities ranging from ordering Preston's meals while he was in the hospital to relaying information to his physicians at home in British Columbia. As she explained, "it's like you go into overdrive, at least for me it was, you went into overdrive." To cope with these responsibilities, she had her adult children, who lived in Canada, assist with liaising with the hospital in Yuma and also in British Columbia to understand Preston's health status and care trajectory. This allowed her to maintain focus on providing practical care and emotional support for Preston while he was in the hospital. She also had friends help her with securing accommodations for an extended stay in Yuma and taking care of some necessary personal paperwork. She explained, "you have support and people. You just need to ask, and people will help you." Gertrude said that she regularly helped other members of her community, both at home and in Yuma, with small tasks and care responsibilities and thus felt that it was appropriate for her to ask others to help her when she was overwhelmed by caregiving responsibilities so as to not become burned out or experience caregiver burden as a result of Preston's acute health needs.

Gertrude's experience of caring for Preston illustrates an important point, which is that international retirement migrants may form local friendship and support networks that they can draw upon to assist them when providing informal care. Unlike forms of transnational mobility that are shorter in length or typically not recurring (e.g., holiday travel, business trips, physician voluntourism), international retirement migrants often return to a particular destination for many consecutive years and in the process of their extended stays they can form local networks. The opportunity to form new friendships and social networks is, in fact, one of the factors that motivates people to participate in international retirement migration (Casado-Diaz 2006; Pickering et al. 2019). Social participation, community building, and group leisure pursuits are also known to promote health among older people, which is another benefit of this aspect of international retirement migration (Barrett et al. 2012; Brown et al. 2008). For those who need to, international retirement migrants who are practicing informal caregiving may be able to draw upon both distant *and* local communities of support to assist them with managing care responsibilities, which can serve to further protect caregivers' health and wellbeing. This is what Gertrude did, wherein she drew upon distant family networks at home and local social networks in Yuma to assist her with caring for Preston. While there is an established literature about transnational caregiving in the context of family separation and caring remotely for aging parents and the ways in which we can support such caregivers (Brijnath 2009; Krzyżowski and Mucha 2014; Lahaie et al. 2009), there has been relatively little acknowledgment of the fact that informal caregiving may happen in the context of international retirement migration. Gertrude's experience not only shows that such care does indeed take place, but also that the supports that these older travelers may draw on to assist them with their care work can span both home and abroad.

VIGNETTE 4: NORMA AND GARETT

Norma and Garett had spent ten winters in Yuma, traveling there from their home in Eastern Canada. After visiting various warm weather destinations in the United States, they both agreed that Yuma was an ideal place for them to spend their winters as exposure to the warm, dry air "helps with everything" in terms of their health and overall wellbeing. They spent just under six months each year in Yuma, living in a stationary trailer in a community for retirement migrants from Canada and the United States. Garret had multiple chronic health conditions that were managed primarily through medication, including diabetes. Because his health was relatively stable, they felt comfortable spending extended time away from home (including being away from his regular physicians in Canada and the publicly funded health care systems they have access to there). They also felt confident that they could manage extended stays in the United States without needing to access health care there and so opted not to purchase travel health insurance. As Garret told: "yeah, we rely on the Canadian health system to maintain us. No question about it." Norma was always careful to book health care appointments and specialist appointments at home in advance of their return and to plan procedures, such as surgeries, around their travel plans for Yuma. She also made sure that Garret had adequate amounts of insulin for the length of time they were planning to stay in Yuma, both for practical reasons (e.g., avoiding having to find a physician in Yuma to write a prescription) and financial reasons (i.e., the cost of insulin in the United States is significantly higher than in Canada, though it can be purchased more affordably across the border from Yuma in Los Algodones, Mexico if needed).

The ways in which Norma cared for Garret and assisted with managing his diabetes was quite consistent between what she did at home in Canada and what she did while they were in Yuma. Critical care work related to Garret's diabetes management for Norma included all meal planning and food purchases both at home and while in Yuma. While Garret firmly believed in giving himself his own insulin injections instead of asking Norma to do this, Norma's care work in the home and overseeing of their daily schedules and activities enabled him to undertake this task in a routine fashion. Overall, they both had a planning mentality and used a combination of planning and routine-making to assist with managing Garret's diabetes. He strongly believed that all international retirement migrants should "plan ahead before you leave. Plan before your trip. Make sure that you organize it in advance." Similarly, they also planned for their return to Canada through booking medical appointments in advance and aligning return-to-home dates with insulin availability. Overall, while their approach to planning included a number of essential items or issues, important ones for Norma's care work related to maintaining their health and managing Garret's diabetes while abroad and at home in a continuous fashion.

Norma and Garret both found comfort in routine and planning. As a care strategy, Norma used consistency in her care work to assist Garret with managing his diabetes. This included taking on the same care responsibilities both at home and abroad, such as grocery shopping, meal planning, managing medications, and scheduling health care appointments. Although there are many transnational practices that may completely disrupt formal or informal care routines (e.g., Spitzer et al. 2003), in the context of international retirement migration by Canadians who travel to the southern United States, Norma's experience shows that consistency and routine are possible. The creation of routines can be very important for coping with caregiving responsibilities as they allow care recipients to form defined expectations and can also assist with making care tasks more manageable (Burman 2001; Wiles 2003). While formal care networks are disrupted in the context of international retirement migration as care recipients and caregivers spend time outside of their home health care systems and usual care providers, consistency in informal caregiving routines like Norma's may assist with creating some of the continuity discussed in vignette one. In Norma and Garret's case, they relied on recreating the structures they had put in place at home while in Yuma and not stepping outside their normal roles and routines. Their ability to do this likely informed their decision to not purchase travel health insurance and, instead, rely on returning to Canada if unexpected health issues emerged.

VIGNETTE 5: FRANCINE AND ROGER

Francine and Roger were married partners in their eighties who had traveled to Yuma from the Canadian province of Alberta for the last sixteen winter seasons. Both had asthma, Francine had rheumatoid arthritis, and Roger also has lung disease. They returned home from Yuma every five weeks for a three-day period so that Francine could receive treatment for a blood condition she managed. The cost of accessing such treatment out-of-pocket in Yuma was prohibitive and so they found the most cost effective strategy was to fly home so she could access that care in Canada where they—along with other Canadians—had access to publicly funded universal medical care for no payment at the point of service. Returning to Canada every five weeks for Francine's treatment was reflective of their overall mentality toward managing their health while abroad. As Francine explained, "we're very careful. If I start to get sick, we'd just fly home." Francine did, however, take copies of her and Roger's medical records with them to Yuma in the chance they did need to seek health care while abroad.

Although both Francine and Roger had defined health needs, Roger took on a substantial caregiver role as rheumatoid arthritis had limited Francine's mobility in unpredictable ways. She was aware of this, noting that "sometimes I can't do much. Other times I can do quite a bit. But, oh yeah, he helps me a lot." Francine was no longer able to drive, and so Roger oversaw their daily logistics regarding getting around Yuma, purchasing groceries and other needed supplies, and their social activities. They also had friends in Yuma to assist Francine as needed, such as with booking flights or taking her out shopping. Roger had to balance caring for Francine against his own health needs, and specifically managing lung disease. At times the dust and particulate matter in the outdoor air exacerbated his condition, which was something he aimed to avoid. He thus had to factor in the winds and dust, which was ample given the desert dust that regularly blows through Yuma, in order to avoid exacerbating his own health while meeting Francine's care needs.

Roger's experience of providing informal care for Francine while they are in Yuma serves as an important reminder that while older people provide significant amounts of care work (Carmichael and Ercolani 2014), they are also more likely to be co-managing their own personal health needs with caregiving responsibilities given their lifestage (Chen et al. 2015; Torres et al. 2010). While this reality is not unique to caregiving in the context of international retirement migration, it serves as an important dimension of caregiving within this transnational practice because international retirement migrants are older people. Thus, those who are informal caregivers are quite likely to be managing their own chronic and/or acute health conditions. This was seen throughout the vignettes presented here, wherein in several cases the primary caregivers also reported having their own chronic illnesses they needed to manage while in Yuma. For example, Roger had to be careful not to exacerbate his lung disease while going outside to run errands for he and Francine. There is a sizeable established literature about the need to "care for caregivers" and support their health and wellbeing, much of which advocates for the development of interventions that can support caregivers' health (Robinson et al. 2005; Wenger 1990). Such interventions rarely consider mobility and the fact that informal caregivers may be moving around transnationally, such as via international retirement migration. An informational intervention designed to support informal caregivers in medical tourism, which is also a transnational mobility, identified five specific areas of advice for those taking on this role: become an informed health care consumer, assess and avoid exposure to risk, anticipate the care recipient's care needs, familiarize yourself with important logistics, and protect your health (Crooks et al 2017). Given the number of Canadian international retirement migrants, a similar tool targeting the specific needs for informal caregivers in this population would be beneficial.

CONCLUSION

Older people travel abroad as international retirement migrants to create new social networks, live in favorable climates, and experience new cultures, among other reasons (Pickering et al. 2019). In some cases, they participate in this transnational mobility for health promoting reasons or even to live in places where formal health care is more affordable (ibid). While these travelers do not go abroad for the *purpose* of providing informal care, many will end up taking on this role and caring for partners, friends, and others with whom they live or share residential communities. The vignettes shared in this chapter provided examples how this care work is undertaken, by whom, and under what circumstances. Each vignette highlighted a specific dimension of informal caregiving in the context of international retirement migration that is shaped by the transnational elements of this practice. These dimensions were that:

1. international retirement migrants who provide informal care can support facilitating continuity of care between home and abroad through gathering and sharing information and undertaking other knowledge broker tasks;
2. international retirement migrants who provide informal care may not view themselves as caregivers, which may result in them not accessing caregiver supports in the destination (e.g., support groups) that can assist them with coping with particular stressors;
3. international retirement migrants who provide informal care may be able to draw upon support networks *both* at home and in the destination community to assist them with coping with care responsibilities;
4. international retirement migrants who provide informal care may be able to keep routines the same or similar between home and abroad, which can assist with keeping care work manageable and care recipients' expectations realistic; and
5. international retirement migrants who provide informal care are likely to have their own health needs and they may benefit from interventions that assist them with minimizing risks to their health that are tailored to their transnational context.

This list of dimensions is not intended to be exhaustive, but it provides an important initial glimpse into understanding key features of how the transnational context of international retirement migration shapes the practice of informal care.

We view this chapter to be an important starting point to understanding how informal caregiving takes place among international retirement migrants.

While there is a rich tradition of caregiving research in a number of disciplines and these studies have examined many critical facets of caregiving in particular contexts, the way in which it takes place in international retirement migration is heretofore unconsidered. Much additional research is thus needed in order to further understand caregiving practices among international retirement migrants, and specifically studies that can support the creation of interventions aimed at protecting their health and wellbeing in addition to that of the care recipient. Ideally subsequent studies will engage different participant groups given that the caregiver-care recipient dyads we interviewed were comprised of heterosexual marital partners living in Canada who wintered in the same U.S. destination of Yuma and thus reasonably homogenous in nature.

ACKNOWLEDGMENTS

Our fieldwork in Yuma was funded by a Planning Grant awarded by the Canadian Institutes of Health Research. Valorie Crooks holds the Canada Research Chair in Health Service Geographies and a Scholar Award from the Michael Smith Foundation for Health Research.

REFERENCES

Barrett, Anne E., Manacy Pai, and Rebecca Redmond. ""It's your badge of inclusion": The Red Hat Society as a gendered subculture of aging." *Journal of Aging Studies* 26, no. 4 (2012): 527–38.

Brijnath, Bianca. "Familial bonds and boarding passes: Understanding caregiving in a transnational context." *Identities: Global Studies in Culture and Power* 16, no. 1 (2009): 83–101.

Brown, Carroll A., Francis A. McGuire, and Judith Voelkl. "The link between successful aging and serious leisure." *The International Journal of Aging and Human Development* 66, no. 1 (2008): 73–95.

Burman, Mary E. "Family caregiver expectations and management of the stroke trajectory." *Rehabilitation Nursing* 26, no. 3 (2001): 94–99.

Callan, Samantha. "Implications of family-friendly policies for organizational culture: findings from two case studies." *Work, Employment and Society* 21, no. 4 (2007): 673–91.

Carmichael, Fiona, and Marco G. Ercolani. "Overlooked and undervalued: the caring contribution of older people." *International Journal of Social Economics* 41, no. 5 (2014): 397–419.

Carretero, Stephanie, Jorge Garcés, Francisco Ródenas, and Vicente Sanjosé. "The informal caregiver's burden of dependent people: theory and empirical review." *Archives of Gerontology and Geriatrics* 49, no. 1 (2009): 74–79.

Casado-Díaz, María Angeles. "Retiring to Spain: An analysis of differences among North European nationals." *Journal of Ethnic and Migration Studies* 32, no. 8 (2006): 1321–39.

Casey, Victoria, Valorie A. Crooks, Jeremy Snyder, and Leigh Turner. "Knowledge brokers, companions, and navigators: a qualitative examination of informal caregivers' roles in medical tourism." *International Journal for Equity in Health* 12, no. 1 (2013): 1–10.

Chen, Meng-Chun, Kuei-Min Chen, and Tsui-Ping Chu. "Caregiver burden, health status, and learned resourcefulness of older caregivers." *Western Journal of Nursing Research* 37, no. 6 (2015): 767–80.

Cho, Kyoung Hee, Sang Gyu Lee, Byungyool Jun, Bo-Young Jung, Jae-Hyun Kim, and Eun-Cheol Park. "Effects of continuity of care on hospital admission in patients with type 2 diabetes: analysis of nationwide insurance data." *BMC Health Services Research* 15, no. 1 (2015): 107–17.

Coates, Ken S., Robert Healy, and William R. Morrison. "Tracking the snowbirds: Seasonal migration from Canada to the USA and Mexico." *American Review of Canadian Studies* 32, no. 3 (2002): 433–50.

Crooks, Valorie A., and Gina Agarwal. "What are the roles involved in establishing and maintaining informational continuity of care within family practice? A systematic review." *BMC Family Practice* 9, no. 1 (2008): 65.

Crooks, Valorie A., Rebecca Whitmore, Jeremy Snyder, and Leigh Turner. ""Ensure that you are well aware of the risks you are taking…": actions and activities medical tourists' informal caregivers can undertake to protect their health and safety." *BMC Public Health* 17, no. 1 (2017): 1–10.

Dahlborg Lyckhage, Elisabeth, and Berit Lindahl. "Living in Liminality—being simultaneously visible and invisible: caregivers' narratives of palliative care." *Journal of Social Work in End-of-Life & Palliative Care* 9, no. 4 (2013): 272–88.

Desrosiers-Lauzon, Godefroy. "Canadian snowbirds as migrants." *Canadian Issues* (2009): 27–32.

Fast, Janet, and Norah Christine Keating. *Family caregiving and consequences for carers: Toward a policy research agenda.* Ottawa: Canadian Policy Research Networks, Inc. (2000). (URL: http://www.cprn.com/en/doc.cfm?doc=432)

Giesbrecht, Melissa, Valorie A. Crooks, and Allison Williams. "Scale as an explanatory concept: evaluating Canada's Compassionate Care Benefit." *Area* 42, no. 4 (2010): 457–67.

Gillick, Muriel R. "The critical role of caregivers in achieving patient-centered care." *Journal of the American Medical Association* 310, no. 6 (2013): 575–76.

Haas, Heiko. "Volunteering in retirement migration: meanings and functions of charitable activities for older British residents in Spain." *Ageing & Society* 33, no. 8 (2013): 1374–1400.

Haggerty, Jeannie L., Robert J. Reid, George K. Freeman, Barbara H. Starfield, Carol E. Adair, and Rachael McKendry. "Continuity of care: a multidisciplinary review." *British Medical Journal* 327, no. 7425 (2003): 1219–21.

Herd, Pamela, and Madonna Harrington Meyer. "Care work: Invisible civic engagement." *Gender & Society* 16, no. 5 (2002): 665–88.

Krzyżowski, Łukasz, and Janusz Mucha. "Transnational caregiving in turbulent times: Polish migrants in Iceland and their elderly parents in Poland." *International Sociology* 29, no. 1 (2014): 22–37.

Lahaie, Claudia, Jeffrey A. Hayes, Tinka Markham Piper, and Jody Heymann. "Work and family divided across borders: The impact of parental migration on Mexican children in transnational families." *Community, Work & Family* 12, no. 3 (2009): 299–312.

Longino Jr, Charles F., Adam T. Perzynski, and Eleanor P. Stoller. "Pandora's briefcase: Unpacking the retirement migration decision." *Research on Aging* 24, no. 1 (2002): 29–49.

Mainous III, Arch G., Richelle J. Koopman, James M. Gill, Richard Baker, and William S. Pearson. "Relationship between continuity of care and diabetes control: evidence from the Third National Health and Nutrition Examination Survey." *American Journal of Public Health* 94, no. 1 (2004): 66–70.

Marshall, Victor W., Charles F. Longino Jr, Richard Tucker, and Larry Mullins. "Health care utilization of Canadian snowbirds: An example of strategic planning." *Journal of Aging and Health* 1, no. 2 (1989): 150–68.

Mittelman, Mary S., William E. Haley, Olivio J. Clay, and David L. Roth. "Improving caregiver well-being delays nursing home placement of patients with Alzheimer disease." *Neurology* 67, no. 9 (2006): 1592–99.

Murphy, Nancy A., Becky Christian, Deidre A. Caplin, and Paul C. Young. "The health of caregivers for children with disabilities: caregiver perspectives." *Child: Care, Health and Development* 33, no. 2 (2007): 180–187.

Nijboer, Chris, Reike Tempelaar, Mattanja Triemstra, Geertrudis AM van den Bos, and Robert Sanderman. "The role of social and psychologic resources in caregiving of cancer patients." *Cancer* 91, no. 5 (2001): 1029–39.

Pickering, John A.J., and Valorie A. Crooks, "Retirement Migration," In *Encyclopedia of gerontology and population aging*, eds. Gu, Danan, and Matthew E. Dupre, R:1–3. Cham: Springer, 2019. (DOI: https://doi.org/10.1007/978-3-319-69892-2_629-1)

Pickering, John A. J., Valorie A. Crooks, Jeremy Snyder, and Jeffery Morgan. "What is known about the factors motivating short-term international retirement migration? A scoping review." *Journal of Population Ageing* 12, no. 3 (2019): 379–95.

Robinson, Louise, Jill Francis, Peter James, Norma Tindle, Kim Greenwell, and Helen Rodgers. "Caring for carers of people with stroke: developing a complex intervention following the Medical Research Council framework." *Clinical Rehabilitation* 19, no. 5 (2005): 560–71.

Romanow, Roy J. *Building on Values : The Future of Health Care in Canada : Final Report*. Privy Council, Commission on the Future of Health Care in Canada, (2002). Online: https://cwhn.ca/en/node/22841

Shen, Megan Johnson, Manna, Ruth, Banerjee, Smita C, Nelson, Christian J, Alexander, Koshy, Alici, Yesne, Gangai, Natalie, Parker, Patricia A, and Korc-Grodzicki, Beatriz. "Incorporating Shared Decision Making into Communication with Older Adults with Cancer and Their Caregivers: Development and Evaluation of a Geriatric Shared Decision-making Communication Skills Training Module." *Patient Education and Counseling*, (2020): 1–7.

Sisk, Rebecca J. "Caregiver burden and health promotion." *International Journal of Nursing Studies* 37, no. 1 (2000): 37–43.

Spitzer, Denise, Anne Neufeld, Margaret Harrison, Karen Hughes, and Miriam Stewart. "Caregiving in Transnational Context: "My Wings Have Been Cut; Where Can I Fly?"." *Gender & Society* 17, no. 2 (2003): 267–86.

Stajduhar, Kelli I. "Examining the perspectives of family members involved in the delivery of palliative care at home." *Journal of Palliative Care* 19, no. 1 (2003): 27–35.

Sunil, Thankam S., Viviana Rojas, and Don E. Bradley. "United States' international retirement migration: the reasons for retiring to the environs of Lake Chapala, Mexico." *Ageing & Society* 27, no. 4 (2007): 489–510.

Torres, Sussan J., Marita McCabe, and C. A. Nowson. "Depression, nutritional risk and eating behaviour in older caregivers." *The Journal of Nutrition, Health & Aging* 14, no. 6 (2010): 442–48.

Villalobos Dintrans, Pablo. "Informal caregivers in Chile: the equity dimension of an invisible burden." *Health Policy and Planning* 34, no. 10 (2019): 792–99.

Weinberg, Dana Beth, R. William Lusenhop, Jody Hoffer Gittell, and Cori M. Kautz. "Coordination between formal providers and informal caregivers." *Health Care Management Review* 32, no. 2 (2007): 140–49.

Wenger, G. Clare. "Elderly carers: the need for appropriate intervention." *Ageing & Society* 10, no. 2 (1990): 197–219.

Whitmore, Rebecca, Valorie A. Crooks, and Jeremy Snyder. "Exploring Informal Caregivers' Roles in Medical Tourism through Qualitative Data Triangulation." *The Qualitative Report* 24, no. 8 (2019): 1852–65.

Wiles, Janine. "Daily geographies of caregivers: mobility, routine, scale." *Social Science & Medicine* 57, no. 7 (2003): 1307–25.

Chapter 3

Care, Choice, and Cure

Exploring the Logics of Mobility of Patients with Breast Cancer in Italy and France

Cinzia Greco

In this chapter, I explore the intra-national mobility of patients with breast cancer in Italy (in particular, in the regions of Apulia and Emilia-Romagna) and France (in the Île-de-France region) and how such mobilities in two different European contexts are influenced by the logics of care, choice, and cure. The patients I interviewed have both utilized micro-mobilities between different healthcare institutions (some in the public and others in the private sector) and, in Italy, mid-range mobilities that in some cases spanned different regions.

Research on health-related mobility has traditionally focused on two international vectors: Global South to Global North movements in search of treatments not available locally (e.g., Pian 2015), and Global North to Global South movements in search of more affordable treatments, often in a context akin to medical tourism (e.g., Dalstrom 2012, Holliday et al. 2015). However, in recent years there has been an enlargement of the types of health-related mobility considered in the literature, including an increased attention to *intra-national* mobility (Vindrola-Padros 2012, Vindrola-Padros and Brage 2016, Pfister and Vindrola-Padros 2018, Molina and Palazuelos 2014, Edmiston 2018, Greco 2019).

Intra-*regional* health-related mobility has initially been explored in reference to rural areas characterized by limited infrastructures, both in terms of healthcare and transport (e.g., Molina and Palazuelos 2014). Mobility between medical institutions in more resource-rich areas, on the other hand, has mostly been explored in terms of navigation of the healthcare system and health-seeking. The concepts of navigation and health-seeking are explicitly opposed to the earlier concept of doctor-shopping and aim to destigmatize the practice of seeing several doctors (cf. Manderson et al. 2008).

In this chapter, I use the concept of micro-mobility to compare the mobilities between institutions that I observed in France to those observed in Italy, as well as the mobilities between cities and regions of patients in Italy. The choice to analyze together mid-range mobilities, and the circulation between different institutions in a same geographical area, follows a general principle of mobility studies, that is, the need to consider a large number of scales rather than delimiting the analysis to scales of mobility that have traditionally attracted more attention (Glick Schiller and Salazar 2013). Micro-mobility entails individual mobilization of different kinds of capital, knowledge, and imagination needed even for small-scale mobility, such as taking a bus (Vindrola-Padros and Johnson 2017). The concept can be linked to that of motility, that is, the different forms of capital that actors have available to complete a mobility—regardless of whether such mobility is actually enacted or not (Kaufman et al. 2004). The concept of micro-mobility has been used to explore how children (Vindrola-Padros and Johnson 2017) navigate the healthcare services with limited resources, in some case creating for themselves the needed resources; and also how transgender people in rural regions of the United States navigate healthcare services that are not tailored for them—and are in some cases hostile, even dangerous (Edmiston 2018).

The women I interviewed in Italy had access to well-developed healthcare services and reasonably developed transport services, although less so in Southern Italy. The motivations behind mobility were mostly looking for an institution they felt they could trust, with further needs to find medical professionals who were more attentive and caring. For the women I interviewed in Île-de-France—an area in which both healthcare and public transport are highly developed—the reasons to move were linked to the need to find more caring medical professionals, but also being able to choose the preferred treatment options.

The different reasons behind health-related mobilities can be explored through the concept of "logic," as defined by Annemarie Mol (2008). Mol has discussed treatments for diabetes in terms of a logic of choice—prioritizing patients' choices, autonomy and responsibility—and of a logic of care—the practical pursuit of patient's well-being, without necessarily asking patients to explicitly choose between distinct treatment options. Andersen and Vedsted (2015) have suggested that reduced resources for, and managerialization of, healthcare have promoted a logic of efficiency that aims to triage patients according to the clarity of their symptoms. Elsewhere (Greco 2019), I have observed that health-related mobility research has mostly been concerned with a logic of access—people moving to access treatments that are not available, or are expensive, locally (e.g., Kangas 2002, Dalstrom 2012), and also a logic of healing—mobility to access practices and areas that could have a healing effect beyond biological efficacy, including therapeutic landscapes (e.g., Williams 2010, Parkin 2010). I suggested that other health-related mobility follows also a logic of cure, that is the search for biological efficacy of biomedical treatments, in particular by choosing the institutions and the doctors considered most capable (Greco 2019—see also Chee and Whittaker 2020 for an analysis of international medical travel that can be linked to a logic of cure). The logic of care, which I include in the current analysis, has also been linked to medical travel in literature, in reference to receiving more attention, information, and empowerment from medical professionals (see, e.g., Speier 2016: 84–89; Vindrola-Padros 2019: 107–111), and to cultural proximity between patients and doctors, particularly in the case of return medical travel (Inhorn 2011).

In this chapter, I examine the logics of healthcare mobility in different geographical contexts, as well as their intersections with the logics of choice and care discussed by Mol. While I identify instances of logics of cure, care, and choice in the stories of my interviewees, I found less relevance for the logic of healing—that is, less evidence that patients sought subjective rather than biological/biomedical solutions to their illnesses. Some interviewees, particularly in Italy, did see their illness experience and recovery, for example, in religious terms, but, in these cases, the logic applied was not linked to mobility of any kind.

The different logics I explore here are to a degree, as with most conceptualizations, ideal types that co-exist in specific cases and often blur one into the other in concrete examples. Starting from studies of cancer diagnoses, MacArtney et al. (2020) have recently suggested that a conceptualization of the doctor–patient relationship that sees agreement and conflict as not mutually exclusive, can be used to see as compatible not only the logic of choice and the logic of care, but also the two logics with medical authority. However, my approach in this chapter is rather to highlight how conflict between the medical system and the patients—something that many of the patients I met have experienced, and expressed, in significant ways—can introduce specific logics to health-related mobility.

The doctor–patient encounter has long been recognized as marked by class and status asymmetries (Waitzkin 1979), and the managerialization of healthcare has emphasized the triage dimension of the relations between patients and healthcare professionals (Anderson and Wedsted 2015). If we look at the larger experience of patients with the medical system, the sequence of the encounters a patient has can trace complex pathways characterized by a difficulty in accessing treatments. Such difficult pathways have been particularly recognized for patients trying to obtain diagnoses for conditions that have limited medical recognition, such as chronic fatigue syndrome (Åsbring and

Närvänen 2004), or that are routinely under-diagnosed, such as endometriosis (Manderson et al. 2008). However, accessing specific treatments post-diagnosis can also be complicated, as my interviewees discovered in the case of a mostly elective treatment such as breast reconstruction.

In the following pages, I first present the healthcare systems of Italy and France and their implications for health-related mobility. After discussing the methods employed, I then analyze in turn the data collected in Italy and in France. I show how the women I met in Italy utilized long- and mid-range mobilities linked to a logic of cure—accessing the most effective treatments, and micro-mobilities linked to logics of cure and of care—being treated by doctors who were attentive and trustworthy. The women I interviewed in France conducted micro-mobilities across public and private institutions, following logics of care and of choice—in particular, they aimed to obtain specific reconstructive techniques. In the final pages, I present conclusions on the resources needed for mobilities and the continuing asymmetries of power between doctors and patients, as well as some reflections of the implications of the recent COVID-19 pandemic for health-related mobilities.

THE ITALIAN AND FRENCH HEALTHCARE SYSTEMS

Italy and France are both countries with advanced, universalistic healthcare systems: Italy has a single-payer healthcare system, inspired by the British National Health Service (NHS), while France has a social insurance system. The difference between the two models consists in the fact that a single-payer system is funded through general taxation and open to the whole population, while a social insurance system is based on compulsory non-profit insurances that refund the health expenses of those contributing to the insurance and of their families (see, e.g., Wendt 2009). In France, there is an atypical social insurance system: there is a single national health insurance that is significantly subsidized by general taxation; those unable to contribute to the social insurance (e.g., because of unemployment) are covered by public insurance schemes, and in most cases treatment costs are covered immediately by insurance rather than refunded in a second moment (Steffen 2010). The implications of the two models for patients can be best understood by looking at the different role of private healthcare, which remains highly relevant in both countries. As the Italian public healthcare system is inspired by the free-at-the-point-of-use norm (with the exception of the *"ticket sanitario,"* the equivalent of a user fee for a number of interventions and for people earning above a certain minimum income), private health insurance has a limited diffusion in Italy. Private healthcare is usually accessed by paying out-of-pocket—although there is also a large use of private provisions of public healthcare (in which case the private institutions are accessed freely by the patients and the cost is covered by the public). In France, both public and private healthcare costs are refunded by the public health insurance, although private providers usually charge above the maximum cost refunded by the public insurance (an approach called *dépassement d'honoraires*). As a result of this insurance-based system, there is a larger use in France of integrative, private healthcare insurances, mostly in the form of non-profit mutual societies (cf. Steffen 2010). In both Italy and France, the use of private healthcare is motivated by the aim to bypass long waiting times in public healthcare, and in some cases by questions of choice, and is stratified according to income. However, the French insurance-based approach tends to stimulate more the use of private healthcare.

Neither country is free from significant inequalities in healthcare (which are stronger along the North/South divide in Italy, in part because of the recent regionalization of the system—see Toth 2014, and for the experiences of the patients, Greco 2019). However, most treatments for breast cancer are available free of cost, or with limited costs, in both countries. Further, neither Italy nor France have significant referral systems for patients wanting to see a specialist, as this is generally a guaranteed right. This means that patients in Italy and France are not generally subject to the mobility barriers represented by the referral system. Even in other advanced universalistic healthcare systems, such as the British and Danish systems, the need to obtain a referral from a general practitioner in order to see a specialist introduces forms of rationing of specialist healthcare (see, e.g., Bevan and Brown 2014, Andersen and Vedsted 2015), as well as limiting the choice of which doctors and in which public healthcare institutions the patient can access. Both Italy and France have specialized institutions for the treatment of cancer (usually publicly funded but regulated by private law), but the French network of such institutions, called Centres de lutte contre le cancer (CLCC—literally "Centers for the fight against cancer") is more developed.

Reconstructing Healthcare Mobilities:
A Note on Methodology

This chapter is based on a research I conducted between 2012 and 2014 in France and in Italy on the experiences of breast cancer, and in particular on breast surgery and post-mastectomy reconstruction. During my fieldwork, I interviewed both medical professionals and patients, including several involved in patients' associations.

In this chapter, I focus particular on in-depth interviews that I have conducted with women with breast cancer, fifty-two in France and twenty-eight in Italy. In France I conducted fieldwork in the Île-de-France region, which includes Paris and is both the richest region in the country and the seat of the most important oncological institutions. In Italy I conducted fieldwork in Apulia in Southern Italy, and in Emilia-Romagna in Northern Italy. There is a significant economic inequality between the richer North and the poorer South in Italy (cf. Greco 2019), and the hospitals in Emilia-Romagna are more prestigious than the ones in Apulia, although arguably the main oncological centers in Italy are located in the Lombardy region, also in the North. I contacted patients through the mediation of doctors and associations and, in Apulia, through my personal networks; from the initial contacts I reached other patients through the snowball procedure. The interviewees were mostly middle-class in France and Northern Italy, with more working-class interviewees in Southern Italy.

Interviews with the patients aimed to reconstruct their illness experience and included questions on the diagnosis, the treatments they underwent and their relationships with the medical personnel. Most interviews were audio recorded with the consent of the patients; when the patients preferred not to be recorded, I took extensive notes during and after the interview. The interviews were conducted in French and in Italian and the extracts here presented are my translations. All the names used are pseudonyms and some minor details have been changed in order to protect the privacy of interviewees. In many cases, the mobility narrations I analyze here were presented spontaneously by the interviewees without a specific question on my part prompting the topic of mobilities. In many cases, the patients themselves highlighted the fact that they moved from one region to another, or from one institution to another, or to have met several doctors before finding one that suited their needs. This underlines the importance of mobilities and micro-mobilities in the experiences of patients with breast cancer.

The analysis is based on systematic comparison across the interviews and between the data collected in France and in Italy. I follow the extended case method (Burawoy 1991) to contextualize the ethnographic data, linking them to structural phenomena at a larger scale than the one observed, and I compare the results with previous literature in order to identify the ways in which the data here deviate from existing theories. This comparative dimension is useful in highlighting the role of the logics of choice, cure, and care in orienting the different mobilities.

Between the Logics of Cure and Care: Mobilities in Italy

Mobility to access healthcare is a common experience in Italy, and it overlaps with historical and current asymmetries of power, financial stability, and prestige between Northern and Southern Italy, the South perceived to be backward when compared with the industrial and rich North (see, e.g.,

Schneider 1998). People living in the South are used to moving to the North to work or to study (cf. Gallo 2015), and health-related internal migrations represent just one of the many internal migrations that characterize Italy.[1] These movements are also linked to differences in healthcare quality (though these are difficult to quantify). In Lombardy, where some of the women I interviewed went for treatment, there are prestigious medical institutions that specialize in the treatment of cancer. However, interviews conducted with patients with breast cancer living both in the North and in the South of Italy have shown that patients in the North also moved to another province or region[2] in order to receive treatments for breast cancer, and in particular in order to undergo the initial surgery. Treatments for breast cancer are available on the whole Italian territory and follow national guidelines—there are no significant treatments for early stage breast cancer that are not available in most oncology departments. This means that these mobilities are not linked to a logic of access, as in other cases of intra-national mobility, in which the treatments are available only in a few locations within the national territory (cf. Vindrola-Padros 2012).

The reason most commonly given for this mobility was the search for competent and trustworthy institutions and doctors. Such logic was fully within the biomedical focus on the biological efficacy of treatments, rather than linked to other principles of healing (cf. the logic of healing described in the introduction above), or to larger considerations of the care experience. Mobility in these cases aims to maximize the opportunities offered by biomedicine. Given the difficulty in defining the success of treatments, and in particular the probabilistic results of all cancer treatments—in which "no evidence of disease" is the best possible result—the trustworthiness of the institution acts as a proxy for biological efficacy. However, this maximization of opportunities is conducted differently between the North and the South of the country. As mentioned, migrations from the South to the North of Italy are considered normal, and there are two consequences of such normalization. Firstly, interviewees I met in Southern Italy perceived undergoing treatment in another province still within the South as being treated locally, as they have not moved to the North for treatments. To the contrary, interviewees in the North who traveled a comparable distance within Northern Italy described the mobility as "going outside the territory" (as Claudia, an interviewee resident in Emilia Romagna and treated in Lombardy and Tuscany, described her own pathway). Secondly, some of the interviewees in the South who were treated locally somehow felt the need to justify their immobility, often by invoking reasons similar to those who moved North, in terms of competence and trustworthiness of the local doctors.

These long- and mid-range intra-national mobilities required different forms of capital (cf. Kaufman et al. 2004; Vindrola and Johnson

2017)—economic (e.g., for travel and accommodation), cultural, as well as social (to identify the institutions and the doctors in which to be treated, but also in some case to rely on family for accommodation). Claudia, the interviewee mentioned above, relied on the advice of friends to identify a surgeon in Pisa for treatments that she could trust to be capable. But even micro-mobilities between medical institutions required specific forms of capital. For many of my interviewees in Southern Italy "knowing the doctor" was even more important. Information that patients can gather by mobilizing their network of family and friends can influence whether and how they decide to move and to change their therapeutic pathway. Luciana, for instance, who at the time of the interview was in her fifties and living in Apulia, told me that she decided to be treated locally because in her province there were good institutions and it was just a matter of finding them. Indeed, she believed that "sometimes we have excellent doctors here and we just don't know it."

Knowing the doctor should not be considered as necessarily having a personal relationship; rather, the possibility of collecting information allows the patients to trust their doctors. This aspect is clarified in Apollonia's story. A woman in her seventies at the time of the interview, she told me of her experience with her breast cancer diagnosis a few years before. Apollonia followed the recommendation of her sister when choosing a doctor to undergo fine needle aspiration biopsy, as the same doctor had treated a friend of her sister years before. When the biopsy presented problems and she was unsatisfied with the first doctor, she tried to rely on other forms of social vicinity when choosing the surgeon to be operated.

> He [the surgeon] had his wife that was from [Apollonia's town]. When he heard people from [that town] he gave particular attention. [. . .] For 24 years he was by the professor in the hospital. Then he went to emergency surgery and said "you have to give attention to everybody, but when people from [Apollonia's town] come you have to treat them well." "So you are from [that town]," people said, "then don't worry."

In some cases, interviewees who did not have the appropriate specialist close to their social network felt they lacked an important resource and were eager to obtain recommendations from the doctor that diagnosed them, as shown in the two excerpts below, taken from the interviews with Celeste and Doriana.

> They give me this [the mammogram], she [the radiologist] says me "look, Madam, as soon as you get out of here go urgently to a surgeon." "A surgeon," I say, "why?" "Because, it's good you are seen by a surgeon." "*Mamma mia*, I really don't know any." She named me more than one. (Celeste)

And then she [the radiologist] told me "look," she says, "you have to be operated as urgently as possible," and I did not know anyone. I said "Doctor," I say, "at least recommend me [. . .] I don't know which way I should turn [. . .]. She says "look, don't worry, now I'll write you a note and you go directly to Dr. ——." (Doriana)

There are two logics behind this need to have a recommendation in order to choose a doctor. Partly, as in case of Apollonia, establishing some social link with the doctor is considered a guarantee one will not receive sub-par treatment. More importantly, the recommendation is considered a way to identify a doctor that is competent, and this aspect is part of a logic of cure.

It is worth emphasizing that in Italy (as in France), patients have more choice in deciding which doctor they should consult. Patients can circulate throughout the national territory and seek treatments where they prefer more freely than in other countries (e.g., in the UK). In Doriana's and Celeste's narratives, it is indeed the patients who ask their radiologists to suggest a surgeon they could contact. This freedom means that patients have to define their own micro-mobilities, including in some cases choosing different institutions for different moments in their therapeutic pathways—diagnosis, surgery, chemotherapy, and so forth. In this context, this kind of knowledge about trustworthy doctors and institutions, derived from their social capital, is part of the resources mobilized to assure such micro-mobility, and can act as a thread that helps patients to orient themselves in a complex healthcare system.

Choice and Care: The Logics behind Micro-Mobility in France

Many of the patients I interviewed in France had experiences of medical mobility within the Île-de-France and between different kinds of healthcare institutions. These experiences confirm Vindrola and Johnson's observation that "in many ways, micro-mobility is both material and symbolic" (2017: 296). The micro-mobilities of my interviewees not only cover different kinds of medical institutions—university hospitals, CLCCs, private clinics—but cast a light on the resources, knowledge, and difficulties that allow or hinder such mobility. For many interviewees, it was the moment of the post-mastectomy reconstruction that interrupted a pathway started within a single institution, pushing them to navigate a complex therapeutic and institutional landscape. Chloé, a woman in her sixties at the time of the interview, told me how, after a complex diagnostic process that went on for years, she finally had the confirmation that the lump in her breast was malignant. Chloé underwent a mastectomy (a total ablation of the breast) followed by radiotherapy and hormonotherapy, and could not have an immediate (contextual to the mastectomy) reconstruction.

Obtaining the reconstruction technique Chloé preferred was difficult, and the woman began moving between different surgeons and different institutions, negotiating with them the kind of technique she wanted. Chloé told me of her discussions with several friends and acquaintances who had had breast cancer, and was able to resort to their experiences; moreover, she was already well informed and had attended medical meetings and conferences. Together, these helped her to define what she hoped for from a reconstruction, but at the same time made her relationship with the medical system more complex: she told me "I think I am a nuisance [*une enquiquineuse*] for the doctors, because I ask loads of questions." Chloé met three different surgeons in the private sector before finding one who sufficiently inspired her confidence, and with whom she underwent the intervention. Different factors oriented her choice, firstly the trust in the operating surgeon:

> [I asked] "what is the difference if it's you [that does the operation]" and he said me "well, —— is a university hospital, so a formation center, and so I'm not the one operating, it's my assistants, but I am there, while if it's at the clinic, I'm the one operating," so evidently, I choose the option, let's say luxury, to be operated by this doctor in the private clinic.

A second important factor was the kind of relation with the medical personnel that the private institution allowed. Chloé felt that in the private sector she had access to the medical professionals for a longer time and thus could gather more detailed information:

> He answered to the questions I asked on a technical level. For example, for the second operation, I did not understand very well from where he took the tissue for the graft, to redo the areola. He showed me, he had a lesson on his computer and he showed me his lesson.

Chloé was able to mobilize cultural capital—her readings and attendance of medical conferences—her social capital—the friends with whom she could exchange information about the illness, the reconstruction, and the names of doctor and institutions—as well as her economic capital. She recognized that she was in a privileged position, being able to finance a reconstruction in a private clinic. It is important to underline that, though for some patients moving to the private sector was experienced as a choice, for others it was the opposite of choice. Many women had their reconstruction in the private sector only because of the long waiting lists in the public one, or, in some cases, upon suggestions by surgeons to move the operation from a public to a private institution. For some of the patients this meant having to pay significant sums out-of-pocket (Greco 2015).

Chloé was not the only patient to utilize micro-mobilities spanning the public and the private sectors. Bénédicte, a patient also in her sixties, following the advice of her gynecologist, and after the diagnosis went to a private institution for her treatment. She considered her gynecologist's advice to be good, as the private clinic allowed her to be treated more rapidly. However, the experience itself was negative. Bénédicte's family history suggested she had an at-risk profile, and she preferred to undergo a dual mastectomy, but the doctor who treated her was opposed to this and agreed to perform the dual mastectomy only after a struggle on Bénédicte's part. Moreover, Bénédicte told me how, after the mastectomy, she "got a nosocomial infection" and "I was treated [*soignée*] badly in the clinic . . . they changed nurses every couple of days, so the nurses made errors when taking out the drains." When she was diagnosed with a local relapse, disappointed by the low quality of care and attention she found in the clinic despite the clinic's good reputation, Bénédicte decided to continue treatments in a public hospital.

Chloé and Bénédicte show a circulation between the public and the private system; Brigitte, a woman in her late fifties at the time of the interview, moved between different public institutions, more precisely between two different CLCCs located in Île-de-France. She underwent her initial operation and the following therapies in one CLCC in the Île-de-France region. The CLCC was not particularly close to her home—she needed 40 to 50 minutes to reach it, even though, as she emphasized, some appointments were only for a 10-minute consultation with a doctor. Brigitte described a difficult relationship in which she could not have good communication with the personnel of the center and felt that her needs were not adequately considered. When she was diagnosed with a relapse in the contralateral breast, the situation worsened. The surgeon that first operated her did not have space in his schedule and sent her to another colleague in the same institution. Brigitte was very disappointed by this behavior but tried to schedule a consultation with the new doctor. In the meantime, she was participating to a project promoted by a patients' association and, in that context, met a volunteer who collaborated with several doctors. The volunteer took interest in Brigitte's case and, as Brigitte did not have a relationship of trust with the doctors who had her in treatment, she advised her to contact a surgeon working in another CLCC. Brigitte was able to get rapidly a consultation with this surgeon and, having more trust in the new doctor, decided to change institutions. These experiences show a mobility that follows the logic of care: patients indeed move to find institutions and professionals that can be trustworthy and attentive.

For other patients, negotiating access to specific treatments, particularly reconstructive techniques, was also an important factor of micro-mobility, and the movements were, in this case, oriented by a logic of choice. Laure, a woman in her forties, discovered a relapse of her breast cancer that made a mastectomy necessary. For Laure, it was important to have a reconstruction as soon as possible, but things went otherwise. She told me how, once she had been discharged from the mastectomy, she found it difficult to obtain information:

> In the hospital in which I has treated there were no reconstructive surgeons and they just said me "Bah, we will put you in prostheses" [. . .] And so I felt a complete void, he [the doctor] wrote me on a small piece of paper, all torn, the names of three plastic surgeons and said me "you can go there, there and there."

The first consultation did not go well at all, so Laure took her "small piece of paper, all torn" and went to the second surgeon and the third. Laure was not satisfied with the proposals of the other two surgeons either, as each of them proposed her either to insert implants or a reconstruction with a self-transplant from the latissimus dorsi muscle. While self-transplant reconstruction is usually preferred to implants because of the more "natural" look that can be obtained, the latissimus dorsi is not the most preferred option, and entails having long-term pain in one's back. At that point Laure started "looking on her own" for information, in particular online. She decided to try with university hospitals, considering that, as in these places "one does research," she could perhaps find a solution. She went to a consultation with a surgeon who proposed that she undergo a DIEP reconstruction. DIEP is another self-transplant technique that uses skin, fat, and blood vessels rather than muscle, is more preferred for aesthetic results, and has fewer side effects, but is also much more complex in terms of time and skill required from the surgeon. After spending a year on a waiting list, Laure found again the kind of body she had been looking for.

This paragraph presents illness trajectories that, while strongly anchored in the individual illness experiences, are not exceptional, but illustrate the different forms of circulation between different public and private institutions—university hospitals, CLCC, private clinics—and between different medical professionals. The two logics proposed by Mol (2008) (i.e., choice and care) intersect in the motivations of these micro-mobilities. On one hand, the patients were looking for good care—timely access to treatments, and the will on the part of medical professionals to offer listening, attention, and communication. While economic capital and the possibility to choose the costlier private institutions could seem to be the key factor in these micro-mobilities, social and cultural capital were also important, and in some cases brought patients to move from the private to the public sector, as in the case of Bénédicte. However, other factors of micro-mobility were linked to the logic of choice—obtaining a dual mastectomy rather than just the mastectomy of the breast with a tumor, as in the case of Bénédicte, and, in several cases, accessing a specific reconstructive technique. I found, both from the illness narratives of patients and from interviews with surgeons, that this choice is often opposed by many surgeons, who see the choice of the technique as purely technical and dependent upon the surgical case, rather than on the preferences of the patient (Greco 2016—see also Greco 2018 on how such attitudes extend to cosmetic surgery). Similarly to the case of patients with endometriosis interviewed by Manderson et al. (2008), for many of my interviewees finding a surgeon willing to use a specific technique was often complex, and the linked illness narratives took specific forms, such as that of the quest, of combat, or of negotiation (Greco 2020).

Logics of Mobility and Breast Cancer: A Provisional Conclusion

The experiences of the patients I met in Italy and France show how the need to move for health reasons is defined along the lines of pre-existing territorial inequalities, as well as according to the capital—economic, social, and cultural—of the patients. Patients use the resources they have available to move within short, medium, or long ranges and, through such mobilities, either aim to extend the opportunities offered by biomedicine (cure), to be able to choose specific treatments, or to receive better care. In the interviews I conducted in Italy I found a greater variety of mobilities. Some patients, who felt the need and had the resources, moved from the South to the North of the country, mainly following the logic of cure, that is, looking for a context in which they could receive the treatments they considered more valid and could be treated by medical professionals they considered more competent and who they could trust. However, there have also emerged kinds of mobility different from those on the South–North axis. In particular, mid-range and micro-mobilities were motivated both by the search for reliable treatments, and for medical professionals who could offer care to the patients, treating them with attentiveness and respect. There is an overlap, in this case, between the logics of care and cure, as for many patients the doctor who is attentive to the patient is also considered more competent, and better able to provide effective treatments. The overlap between the two logics is often linked to the fact that patients consider an attentive and caring doctor to also be a doctor who can give the patients a better access to the possibilities of biomedicine. This includes treatments or surgical techniques that can be more complex, but have less side effects or are less invalidating.

The patients I interviewed in France conducted mainly important micro-mobilities between different medical institutions, in particular micro-mobilities from the public to the private sector and vice versa. In some cases, given the long and complex pathway linked to a disease such as breast cancer, there is a co-presence of the two sectors—for example, continuing follow-up consultations in the public sector but having breast reconstruction in the private one. These micro-mobilities are linked to a logic of choice—finding the medical professional with whom one can have a specific treatment, such as a specific surgical technique for breast reconstruction—as well as to a logic of care—for example, looking for more listening from medical professionals. In some cases, looking at the micro-mobilities allows to emphasize the emotional layers of the doctor–patient relationship. For some patients being listened and considered in their individuality was a very important aspect, as the case of Laure shows. Being listened was a way for the patient to feel that doctors were offering care to them as a person and not simply to a body district affected by cancer.

In the experiences of both Italian and French patients, motility (i.e., the capacity for movement) relies on the specific relevant organization of the public healthcare sector, that is, on not being limited in the choice of medical institution by the place of residence (the so-called "postcode lottery,"—c.f. Russell et al. 2013) nor by rigid systems of referral (e.g., those existing in the UK and in Denmark). Regardless of whether the patients decide to be treated locally or elsewhere, the capacity to choose—and the motility expressing this capacity—is also a resource when the dominant logic is one of cure or care. However, patients are more explicit in defining their mobility in terms of choice when micro-mobility involves the private sector. Most interviewees who included the private sector in their therapeutic pathway have done so when undergoing a breast reconstruction. Such intervention, however, often comes months if not years after the end of curative therapies. Such temporality, separated from the urgency of other treatments, in particular the surgery to remove the tumor, also facilitates the circulation between different medical professionals and institution in search of the best option. In this sense, the neoliberal dimension of the logic of choice highlighted by Mol (2008) is expressed in the fact that the micro-mobilities toward the private sector follow the assumptions of the consumerist power in the context of market choice (the logic of care however is not incompatible with neoliberal/consumerist medical travel—see Speier 2016). The fact that this choice manifests in consumerist terms, however, is also a reflection of the asymmetry in the doctor–patient relationship, further accentuated by the gender asymmetry between women patients and predominantly male surgeons. Despite the formal democratization of the doctor–patient relationship (see, e.g., Rothman 2001), patients still have difficulty obtaining the kind of treatment they prefer even in a substantially elective case such as post-mastectomy reconstruction. If democratization was substantial and women could successfully negotiate the kind of technique with most surgeons, there would be less need for a consumerist search for options on the market. However, most of these choices are exercised through micro-mobility between different medical professionals, in search of the one capable and willing to use the desired technique, rather than in the relation and the negotiation with a specific surgeon.

The Uncertain Future of Mobility: A Post-scriptum

The writing of this chapter was finalized between March and April 2020, while most countries were in unprecedented situations of lockdown introduced to reduce the spread of the COVID-19 disease. At the moment of writing (April 2020), mobility is drastically reduced, including in Italy and France, and limited to essential activities such as buying food or medicines and for essential healthcare treatments. Further, even the health mobilities that can be conducted during the lockdowns and the pandemic are extremely limited: elective and non-essential treatments have often been cancelled across medical institutions. These limitations to mobility particularly affect patients with cancer. "Given the susceptibility of patients with cancer to SARS-CoV-2 infection, their presence at hospitals should be minimized," is the message of the French guidelines published in Lancet Oncology (You 2020: 619), and in many cases doctors and patients have to make difficult decisions on how to manage therapies with the risk of COVID-19. At the moment of writing, the kind of mobilities analyzed in these pages cannot take place either in Italy or in France, which entails inconveniences and uncertainties among patients. There is further uncertainty regarding how the transition to end these lockdowns will be introduced, but there are reasons to think that the return to the status before the pandemic will be gradual and the many limitations will remain for a long time. One would imagine that the mobility of patients with cancer will be altered for the immediate future. The current situation, which saw a rapid reorganization of healthcare services, allows us perhaps to understand another side of mobility—that is, its precariousness.

For many of the patients I met, moving was a need in order to receive the kind of treatments and care they considered important, to be able to conduct some kind of negotiation with the medical system, and to deal with the asymmetries inherent in the doctor–patient relationships. The motility resources they had to use are only partially effective and are, even in the best of times, available only to some of the patients, and can become almost completely useless in situations such as the lockdowns currently imposed on patients' pathways. From within the pandemic, we see further how the motility involved in the cases analyzed here is linked to the unequal distribution of resources. We can see also how the mobilities presented are the result not only of the freedom of choice within healthcare systems, but also of the inequalities within the same systems, which in some cases can be circumvented through mobilities that construct complex therapeutic pathways. In a near future in which the resources mobilized by the patients—social relations, public transport, multiple consultations before identifying the right doctors—could disappear, one wonders how this will change the illness experiences. Further, what resources will be mobilized for the logic of care, cure, and choice in the future? There is obviously no answer at the moment for these questions, but they show the importance of healthcare mobilities and the risks linked to their limitation in the future.

NOTES

1. I discuss mid-range mobilities in Italy in more detail in Greco 2019.
2. Regions are the first level administrative subdivisions in Italy, and are further subdivided in provinces and municipalities.

REFERENCES

Andersen, Rikke Sand and Peter Vedsted. 2015. "Juggling efficiency. An ethnographic study exploring healthcare seeking practices and institutional logics in Danish primary care settings." *Social Science & Medicine*, 128: 239–245.

Åsbring, Pia and Anna-Liisa Närvänen. 2004. "Patient power and control: A study of women with uncertain illness trajectories." *Qualitative Health Research*, 14(2): 226–240.

Bevan, Gwyn and Lawrence D. Brown. 2014. "The political economy of rationing health care in England and the US: the 'accidental logics' of political settlements." *Health Economics, Policy and Law*, 9(3): 273–294.

Burawoy, Michael. 1991. "The Extended Case Method." In *Ethnography Unbound: Power and Resistance in the Modern Metropolis*, edited by Michael Burawoy et al., 271–209. Berkeley, CA: University of California Press.

Chee, Heng Leng and Andrea Whittaker. 2020. "Moralities in international medical travel: moral logics in the narratives of Indonesian patients and locally-based facilitators in Malaysia." *Journal of Ethnic and Migration Studies*, 46(20): 4264–4281.

Dalstrom, Matthew D. 2012. "Winter Texans and the re-creation of the American medical experience in Mexico." *Medical Anthropology*, 31(2): 162–177.

Edmiston, E. Kale. 2018. "Community-led peer advocacy for transgender healthcare access in the Southeastern United States: The trans buddy program." In *Healthcare in Motion: Immobilities in Health Service Delivery and Access*, edited by Cecilia Vindrola-Padros, Ginger A. Johnson and Anne E. Pfister, 185–201. New York: Berghahn.

Gallo, Stefano. 2015. *Senza attraversare le frontiere: Le migrazioni interne dall'Unità a oggi*. Roma-Bari: Laterza.

Glick Schiller, Nina and Noel B. Salazar. 2013. "Regimes of mobility across the globe." *Journal of Ethnic and Migration Studies*, 39(2): 183–200.

Greco, Cinzia. 2015. "The *Poly Implant Prothèse* breast prostheses scandal: Embodied risk and social suffering." *Social Science & Medicine*, 147: 150–157.

———. 2016. "Shining a light on the grey zones of gender construction: breast surgery in France and Italy." *Journal of Gender Studies*, 25(3): 303–317.

———. 2018. "Tailoring the Perfect Patient: Italian Cosmetic Surgeons between Gender Stereotypes and Professional Routines." *AboutGender*, 13 doi: 10.15167/2279-5057/AG2018.7.13.496.

———. 2019. "Moving for cures: Breast cancer and mobility in Italy." *Medical Anthropology*, 38(4): 384–398.

———. 2020. "Quête, combat ou négociation ? Raconter les marges d'action dans le cas de la reconstruction post-mastectomie." *Corps*, 18: 225–234.

Holliday, Ruth et al. 2015. "Brief encounters: Assembling cosmetic surgery tourism." *Social Science & Medicine*, 124: 298–304.

Inhorn, Marcia C. 2011. "Diasporic dreaming: return reproductive tourism to the Middle East." *Reproductive BioMedicine Online*, 23(4): 582–591.

Kangas, Beth. 2002. "Therapeutic itineraries in a global world: Yemenis and their search for biomedical treatment abroad." *Medical Anthropology*, 21(1): 35–78.

Kaufman, Vincent, Manfred Max Bergman, and Dominique Joye. 2004. "Motility: Mobility as capital." *International Journal of Urban and Regional Research*, 28(4): 745–756.

MacArtney, John I. et al. 2020. "The convivial and the pastoral in patient–doctor relationships: a multi-country study of patient stories of care, choice and medical authority in cancer diagnostic processes." *Sociology of Health & Illness*, 42(4): 844–861.

Manderson, Lenore, Narelle Warren, and Milica Markovic. 2008. "Circuit breaking: Pathways of treatment seeking for women with endometriosis in Australia." *Qualitative Health Research*, 18(4): 522–534.

Mol, Annemarie. 2008. *The logic of care: Health and the problem of patient choice*. London: Routledge.

Molina, Rose Leonard and Daniel Palazuelos. 2014. "Navigating and circumventing a fragmented health system: The patient's pathway in the Sierra Madre region of Chiapas, Mexico." *Medical Anthropology Quarterly*, 28(1): 23–43.

Parkin, David. 2014. "Pathways to healing: Curative travel among Muslims and non-Muslims in Eastern East Africa." *Medical Anthropology*, 33(1): 21–36.

Pfister, Anne E. and Cecilia Vindrola-Padros. 2018. "Fluid and mobile identities: Travel, imaginaries, and caregiving practices among families of deaf children in Mexico City." In *Healthcare in Motion: Immobilities in Health Service Delivery and Access*, edited by Cecilia Vindrola-Padros, Ginger A. Johnson and Anne E. Pfister, 77–98. New York: Berghahn.

Pian, Anaïk. 2015. "Care and migration experiences among foreign female cancer patients in France: Neither medical tourism nor therapeutic immigration." *Journal of Intercultural Studies*, 36(6): 641–657.

Rothman, David J. 2001. "The origins and consequences of patient autonomy: A 25-year retrospective." *Health Care Analysis*, 9(3): 255–264.

Russell, Jill et al. 2013. "Addressing the 'postcode lottery' in local resource allocation decisions: a framework for clinical commissioning groups." *Journal of the Royal Society of Medicine*, 106(4): 120–123.

Schneider, Jane, ed. 1998. *Italy's 'Southern Question': Orientalism in One Country*. Oxford: Berg.

Speier, Amy. 2016. *Fertility Holidays: IVF Tourism and the Reproduction of Whiteness*. New York: New York University Press.

Steffen, Monika. 2010. "The French health care system: Liberal universalism." *Journal of Health Politics, Policy and Law*, 35(3): 353–387.

Toth, Federico. 2014. "How health care regionalisation in Italy is widening the North-South gap." *Health Economics, Policy and Law*, 9(3): 231–249.

Vindrola-Padros, Cecilia. 2012. "The everyday lives of children with cancer in Argentina: Going beyond the disease and treatment." *Children & Society*, 26(6): 430–442.

———. 2019. *Critical Ethnographic Perspectives on Medical Travel*. London: Routledge

——— and Eugenia Brage. 2016. "Child medical travel in Argentina: Narratives of family separation and moving away from home." In *Children's Health and Wellbeing in Urban Environments*, edited by Christina R. Engler, Robin Kearns and Karen Witten, 128–144. London: Routledge.

——— and Ginger A. Johnson. 2017. "Children seeking health care: International perspectives on children's use of mobility to obtain health services." In *Movement, Mobilities, and Journeys*, edited by Caitriona Ní Laoire and Allen White, 289–306. Singapore: Springer.

Waitzkin, Howard. 1979. "Medicine, superstructure and micropolitics." *Social Science & Medicine Part A*, 13: 601–609.

Wendt, Claus. 2009. "Mapping European healthcare systems: a comparative analysis of financing, service provision and access to healthcare." *Journal of European Social Policy*, 19(5): 432–445.

Williams, Allison. 2010. "Spiritual therapeutic landscapes and healing: A case study of St. Anne de Beaupre, Quebec, Canada." *Social Science & Medicine*, 70(10): 1633–1640.

You, Benoit et al. 2020. "The official French guidelines to protect patients with cancer against SARS-CoV-2 infection." *The Lancet Oncology*, 21(5): 619–621.

Chapter 4

Providing High Quality Care

What Cross-border Medical Travel Can Teach Us

Matthew Dalstrom

People going to Mexico shows us more about how our system fails us than anything else.

—Texas physician

I was sitting in the front seat of a BMW with Dr. Joe as we drove from his office at a hospital in El Paso, Texas, to a private hospital across the U.S./Mexico border in Ciudad Juarez where he works one or two days a week. Weaving through traffic, he frequently slowed down to point out malls, tourist attractions, and new construction, highlighting how the city has changed since he moved to the area about twenty years ago. Each site had a story that oscillated between his reflections on the drug violence such as when his colleague was kidnapped "right here," to the nostalgic and cosmopolitan aspects of a city that is so often portrayed negatively in the U.S. media. As we approached his hospital, he pivoted and said, "You see people come to Mexico because of the cost, location, and because it is more personalized." In the United States they practice "maquilla medicine," he continued, referring to the assembly plants on the Mexican side of border. "I see close to 80 patients a day in the U.S., but here . . . we spend time with the patients," he explained. Furthermore, working in Mexico gives him the opportunity to talk, develop relationships, and provide "some of the best healthcare in the world." To emphasize his point, he continued, "I had a patient [from the U.S.] who needed a hysterectomy, a nurse, and she was unsure . . . so we talked on the phone about her procedure several times and reviewed her medical records together." Satisfied she went to Mexico to visit him in person, toured the hospital, and he helped her with scheduling the surgery, transferring medical records, and in crossing the border. "We were able to provide the care she needed," he explained, "address her concerns and . . . make her happy."

Curious to understand how his patient interpreted her medical experience, I interviewed her a few weeks later. During our call, Sharron explained how she delayed care in the United States because she was frightened of both the surgery and cost. However, when she saw a news story about medical travel to Mexico, she decided to explore the option. After searching the internet for information, she contacted a medical travel facilitator company that refers patients to Mexican physicians. They provided her with Dr. Joe's contact information and once she decided to call Dr. Joe, she was surprised how easy it was to schedule a time to talk, how personal he was, and how the entire level of care was superior to anything that she had experienced in the United States. As she recalled, it was "one of the best experiences as far as nursing care, level of attention, had a private room, the nurses were excellent, you push a button and they are there . . . they didn't cut staffing because they were low on patients, the food was good." Moreover, she had time to talk with Dr. Joe, ask questions, felt listened to, and did not have to worry about unexpected medical bills because the surgery's cost was bundled meaning that the price was set prior to the surgery.

Sharron's story is not unique and illustrates the type of healthcare experience that Americans can receive at private clinics and hospitals in Mexico. It also points to the dissatisfaction that patients have with medical care in the United States, specifically their limited access to high quality, personal, affordable, and timely healthcare, even for those who are insured. However, little is known about how U.S. residents' perceptions of their own medical system and of medical travel shape the type of care that is provided in private clinics, offices, or hospitals in Mexico. Nor is it clear how medical travel facilitators, patients, and medical providers work together to shape the type of care provided. This chapter will explore the types of care that U.S. patients seek in Mexico, the strategies that Mexican medical providers use to provide that care, and how medical travel facilitators articulate, and support the type of care that patients' desire. It will also discuss how patients' experiences with medical travel to Mexico can be used to improve the delivery of healthcare in the United States.

PATIENT EXPERIENCES IN THE UNITED STATES

There have been many attempts to improve the U.S. healthcare system although the most substantial change in the last thirty years has been the passage of the Patient Protection and Affordable Care Act (ACA), in 2010, which was designed to decrease the uninsured rate, control healthcare costs, and improve the quality of care. The ACA partially achieved two of its goals by first reducing the uninsured rate, although it varies between states, and secondly by slowing the growth of some healthcare costs. Nonetheless, the price of purchasing health insurance continues to rise, albeit more slowly, forcing many patients to purchase lower quality health insurance plans (Kaiser Family Foundation 2019). As a result, while the number of uninsured adults has dropped significantly, it has not always translated into improved access to care due to high-deductibles and co-pays, which makes healthcare unaffordable for many adults. Instead as Susan Sered (2018) points out, the ACA has created a "smorgasbord of donut holes, coverage gaps, and nonsensical limits" (174).

The third goal of the ACA was to improve the quality of care though supporting patient-centered approaches that improve patients' experiences and outcomes (Millensen and Marci 2012). The concept of patient-centered care (PCC) was first introduced in the 1950s (Balint 1955) and decades of research has shown that focusing on the social, emotional, and educational needs of the patient improves both their health, and satisfaction with the care received (Moerman 2002; Wolf et al. 2008; Aboumatar et al. 2015). However, PCC did not become popular in the United States until after the Institute of Medicine published, *Crossing the Quality Chasm: A New Health System for the 21st Century* (2001), which identified PCC as one of the six important strategies to improve the U.S. healthcare system (McKinney 2011). According to the report, PCC entails, "providing care that is respectful of and responsive to individual patient preferences, needs, and values and ensuring that patient values guide all clinical decisions" (Institute of Medicine 2001: 6). PCC has been interpreted in many ways, but regardless of how PCC strategies are implemented into the clinical setting, they generally include an emphasis on shared decision-making, understanding the patient's perspective, asking open-ended questions (Hashim 2017), and are guided by patient preferences and needs (Laine 1996) as opposed to the disease-focused biomedical model that undervalues the patient experience (Aboumtheatar et al. 2015). Within the United States, PCC is primarily emphasized during the patient encounter (Dwamena 2012; Finerock et al., 2018); however, some have argued that PCC should expand beyond it to include supporting the transition of care from one healthcare provider to another, coordinating patient care, and offering emotional support (Gerteis et al. 1993, Edgman-Levitan, and Daley et al. 1993).

While most patients report that they want some version of PCC, and research shows that it improves patient outcomes and satisfaction (Dwamena 2012), it is an underused strategy in the United States (Berry 2009). This can be in part attributed to limited provider time, high patient loads, lack of guidelines, and a feeling among health care providers that PCC is not effective or important (Kiwanuka et al. 2019; Berry 2009). It is also because PCC is often at odds with the neoliberal healthcare model in the United States that emphasizes the importance personal decision-making (not shared) and efficiency, which simultaneously shifts the responsibility of care onto the patients and limits the amount of time that patients have with their provider. For the most part, healthcare in the United States is delivered with the assumption that the patient is a rational consumer, knowledgeable about personal healthcare, and if given the right amount of choices they will choose the best care for themselves (Mulligan 2017). Therefore, choice, is perceived to be both a hallmark of good care (Mol 2008) and as a tool to increase patient engagement. The emphasis on the importance of choice has also recast the responsibility of the clinician from one who guides patient decisions to one who expects patients to make their own, becoming what Premji et al. (2014) refer to as "choice brokers." Nevertheless, while many medical providers are champions of expanding choice and see it as a necessary component (Premji et al., 2014), the negative consequences of a market-based approach that emphasizes choice over other care modalities has been reported (Rylko-Bauer and Farmer 2002; Mol 2008).

Research on patient choice has questioned whether patients can choose, make informed decisions and whether they feel that more choice is the best way to receive better care (Dalstrom 2020; Mulligan 2017). Within the United States, much of the responsibility of navigating the healthcare system has shifted from medical providers to patients even though there are few resources available for patients to help them coordinate their care and make wise medical decisions. In practice, this means that patients are expected to select a health insurance plan, medical provider, treatment, and understand how the healthcare system works, although many adults are unprepared to do so (Politi et al. 2014; Mulligan 2017). The problem is further exacerbated because cost-saving measures frequently limit the amount of time providers spend with their patients which undermines their ability to identify patient needs, educate them, and engage in shared decision-making. Instead much of the education is outsourced to post-visit summaries, pamphlets, or websites. Research on the consequences of shifting so much responsibility to the patient and limiting the amount of time that they have with providers has shown that it undermines the relationship between patients and providers, makes the patient feel like they are not being listened to, puts a considerable burden on patients, and leads to complaints that the experience is impersonal (Victoor 2012; Kleinman 2007; Dalstrom 2020). It has also led some medical anthropologists to question whether it is possible to provide appropriate care within the current healthcare infrastructure (Kleinman 2007).

Medical Travel and Patient Preferences

The failure of the U.S. healthcare system to provide affordable, quality care is especially evident among those who feel like they have few options aside from traveling abroad. This practice, commonly referred to as medical travel or in some cases medical tourism, encompasses a wide range of medical procedures such as orthopedic and cardiac surgery, dental work, physician visits, and other types of preventive care (Lunt, Horsfall, and Hanefeld 2016; Sobo 2009). It is estimated that approximately 1.4 million Americans traveled abroad for medical care in 2017 (Dalen 2018) however, if primary care, dental care, and pharmaceuticals are included the number would be much higher.

Exploring the concept of care through the lens of medical travel illustrates how medical travelers and their families balance the difficulties and dangers of seeking treatment with their expectations for care. Traveling for medical care is not only logistically challenging, but potentially poses health risks for patients. For instance, many patients travel without a referral from their primary care provider (Johnston et al. 2011) and, therefore, are responsible for selecting a treatment destination, medical provider, and navigating a foreign health system without any medical guidance. It has been suggested that traveling long distances for care puts medical travelers at an elevated risk for complications during surgery and on their travel back home. Other concerns raised include the transfer of medical records, delivery of postoperative care, and impact on patient-provider relationships (Crooks et al. 2015; Johnston et al. 2011). Nevertheless, according to Beth Kangas (2002), the allure of medical travel "heightens peoples' expectations" that a cure exists (37) and provides hope that they can access the type of care that they want abroad while encouraging them to take that risk. It also highlights how access to care in the United States can be so inadequate that Milstein and Smith (2006) have dubbed medical travelers from the United States as "medical refugees" who are akin to economic refugees in search of healthcare that they can afford.

While there are many factors (e.g., cost, distance, etc.) that patients and families consider when they make the decision to travel, the type of care is always considered. For instance, according to Speier (2016) medical travelers also want emotional and logistic support in addition to quality medical care. In response, many medical providers have incorporated aspects of PCC into the way that they provide care for foreign patients. Although the term PCC is infrequently used in the medical travel literature, many providers and health systems use PCC strategies to attract foreign patients (see Mason 2014; Speier 2016; Inhorn 2018). While there can be a significant amount of diversity as to how medical providers implement these strategies, they often entail reducing barriers to accessing care, incorporating amenities, and focusing on the patient experience before, during, and after the medical encounter. To assist them in providing this type of care, medical providers and health systems often operate a medical travel program or partner with a medical travel facilitator (MTF) company. While the services that these programs and companies offer vary, they primarily focus on advertising, assuaging patient concerns, and arranging care (Dalstrom 2013; Snyder et al. 2011). In many situations MTFs are the initial point of contact for medical travelers (as opposed to medical providers), and if a health system has a medical travel program, it will often work with patients on transferring medical records, arranging surgical consults, and completing the needed paperwork (e.g., insurance claims) (Ormond and Sothern 2012; Chee, Whittaker, and Por 2017).

To understand how the actors (patients, providers, MTFs) interact to shape how care is provided, there is no better place to explore than along the U.S./Mexico border. Mexico is the most popular medical destination for U.S. residents. It is estimated that 37.3 percent of Texas border residents have traveled to Mexico for physician services and 6.7 percent for inpatient care (Su et al. 2011) and *Newsweek* reported that nationally approximately 800,000 U.S. residents use Mexican healthcare (Da Silva 2019). Unlike other locations, the proximity to Mexico, and the relative ease for permanent U.S. residents and citizens to cross the border has made accessing medical care, even primary care in some cases, possible and affordable (at least when compared to the United States). While people can and do travel to major cities around Mexico for medical care, the majority of medical services are located along the U.S./Mexico border in small towns referred to as medical border towns (Oberle and Arreloa 2004).

The types of care that people seek and the reasons why they travel to Mexico can be very diverse. For instance, Bergmark et al. (2008) found that Latinos return for care in Mexico because of unsuccessful treatments in the United States, a preference for Mexican care, or challenges accessing care in the United States. Horton and Cole (2011) also identified that rapid services, personal attention, effective medications, cost, and confidentiality were often reported as reasons for preferring Mexican healthcare. Other research among non-Hispanic adults has shown that cost, type of treatment, perceptions of Mexican providers, and the relationship with Mexican medical providers are also reasons for accessing care (Dalstrom, Chung, and Castronovo 2020; Addams et al. 2017). However, as Horton and Cole (2011) point out, it is not the public healthcare in Mexico that medical travelers want which is associated with long lines, provider shortages, and short patient visits, instead it is a type of care that is practiced at private clinics, many of which who cater to foreign and/or wealthier Mexican patients.

METHODS

Ethnographic data for this chapter were collected through participant observation and semi-structured interviews that were part of three separate studies on cross-border medical care between the United States and Mexico conducted between 2008 and 2017. Participant observation was conducted in three Mexican border cities (Reyosa, Nuevo Progresso, and Ciudad Juarez) at two hospitals, three dental clinics, three pharmacies, and two physician offices. Semi-structured interviews occurred either in person or over the telephone with 100 medical travelers who were identified through snowball sampling, convenience sampling, and the Winter Texan Migrant Panel, which is maintained through the University of Texas Rio Grande Valley. I also traveled to Mexico with fifteen participants as they sought dental care, pharmaceuticals, and primary care. Additional interviews were conducted with six medical travel facilitators, fifteen Mexican medical providers who practiced along the U.S./Mexico border, and twelve medical providers working in Texas.

PATIENTS IN SEARCH OF CARE

Among those I interviewed, the decision to travel to Mexico for healthcare was influenced by a wide array of factors such as class, ethnicity, citizenship, and age. The commonality which occurred across all the cases was that people sought healthcare in Mexico because of the care they received (or in many cases did not receive in the United States). While cost was commonly mentioned as a barrier, the poor/impersonal care that they received in the United States was cited by almost all of the participants. The complaints about the U.S. health system were varied but centered on primarily on how the U.S. healthcare system operated which included long waiting times, high costs, insurance barriers, and restrictions. Many participants mentioned how confusing it was to find out what was covered by their insurance or even the challenges of learning the basics of how to use their health insurance. As one woman explained, "It is harder and harder to afford healthcare and insurance is confusing." Others said that they had to wait months to get an appointment or that insurance barriers prevented them from getting the type of treatment that they needed. Often the challenges of accessing healthcare were interpreted as the healthcare system not caring about them. As one patient explained, "American doctors care less for the patient, they are in it for the money, they don't spend much time with patient, they care less, and make the patient come back for repeat visits."

These experiences were often juxtaposed to the private Mexican healthcare system available to medical travelers, which they felt was less complicated and more caring since they did not have to deal with health insurance, making it easier to navigate. As one patient explained, "I didn't have to worry, without insurance I knew what it was going to cost." Another mentioned that insurance companies "create blockades . . . [and] in the end there is really no other choice but medical tourism." "In Mexico, you wait less time, Mexican medicine is better . . . they have never asked me for insurance you just walk in and pay . . . and you can easily get an appointment," another commented.

Closely linked to their concerns about cost and ability to navigate the healthcare system was the time that medical providers spent with their patients and how those providers cultivated relationships (or not) with them. Reflecting on her last appointment with a primary care provider one patient explained, "Mexican doctors spend more time with me, they actually listen, and therefore their diagnosis is better." Another said, "I feel more human in Mexico, not a number." Others focused on how providers in the United States are not empathetic or consider patient preferences. For example, Maria, a Mexican-American woman in her sixties was born in Mexico and immigrated to the United States shortly after the Vietnam War. As a school employee in Texas she has good health insurance coverage, a reasonable deductible, and a primary care provider in the United States. Her first experience with the U.S. healthcare system was when she had her first child. She recalled,

> I don't like how they treat me. I don't like that they're expensive, impersonal, that they don't practice clinical medicine, before they look me in the eye they say that I am going to do this and that test . . . . So I was asking questions and the doctor said if you go outside, we have a pamphlet there.

Dissatisfied with the experience, she decided to get her prenatal care for her second child in Mexico (at a higher cost) where she felt that they practiced a more holistic type of healthcare and spent more time talking to her.

Aside from their relationship with the Mexican medical provider, medical travelers also mentioned how important the overall experience of seeking and receiving care was for them. As one explained, "Mexican and U.S. healthcare is comparable, the quality, facilities, and equipment . . . the education is comparable . . . . [except] in the U.S. the docs don't want to waste time or money, so quick, the nurses do everything" and the "experience is different [in Mexico]," a medical traveler explained to me. The experience that has was referring to was not just the clinical encounter, or the interaction with the medical provider, but the process of seeking care and the nonmedical aspects of the encounter. This included how he was treated scheduling the appointment, the short waiting time in the office, and the friendly demeanor of the staff which was interpreted as respect and caring. This type of experience where they felt listened to, not rushed, and were treated as a human, as

Speier (2015) explains, empowers patients, reverses the dominant role of the physician, and is emblematic of "caring."

MEDICAL TOURISM FACILITATORS

A commonly cited problem for patients in the United States is the challenge faced in both navigating the healthcare system, selecting medical providers, and in making medical decisions. "It has always struck me as odd that we know more about the hotel we are staying at than the doctor we are going to," the owner of a medical tourism facilitator company explained to me. "Health is extremely personal, and different than other things we buy . . . . people want the best value . . . and they want to know that they will be cared for." However, that is especially difficult in the United States because that information and support is hard to find or unavailable.

Navigating the U.S. healthcare system is challenging at best and impossible at worst. Numerous studies have shown that people across the economic spectrum struggle to understand insurance coverage, access medical providers, understand medical bills, and make medical decisions (Mulligan and Castenada 2017; McCullough and Dalstrom 2018). Since so many people have problems using their own healthcare system, the challenges of using the Mexican healthcare system might seem insurmountable. This is especially true for those individuals who live far away from the border, do not have personal connections to Mexican healthcare, or are unfamiliar with Mexico in general. In these cases, potential patients can turn to medical tourism facilitators (MTFs) which are companies that specialize in providing patients with healthcare information and in navigating the healthcare system. While there is a tremendous amount of diversity between the companies that provide services in Mexico (see Dalstrom 2013), full service MTFs generally work with a select number of Mexican medical providers, help patients arrange appointments, schedule travel, provide them with information, and in some case with filling out any insurance paperwork. A few also advise Mexican medical providers on the type of care U.S. patients want, how to advertise, and the expected office aesthetics. As one MTF reflected on the type of care that American patients want, "their level of expectation is different. Our sense of entitlement is different . . . the American consumer is quite different . . . and [Mexican medical providers] have to be prepared and have some experience working with Americans." So what do American patients want, "customer service . . . not that hierarchical relationship that traditionally exists in the patient-doctor relationship," "to be consumers with choices," "have modern care," and they want the process to be "easy." Therefore, the services offered and the way that Mexican medical providers provide those services must align with those expectations to be successful in attracting patients.

To encourage patients to travel, these companies frequently advertised the quality of care that could be obtained in Mexico through focusing on value or cost, quality (measured by health outcomes), and how they empower patients to make medical decisions. Often this was done through patient testimonials which were seen as the most effective strategy, because it makes potential "patients feel like that can do it too." Furthermore, it lets them know that they can get "world class care" that they can "afford." However, claiming that care is good, is not enough because healthcare is a personal experience and each patient has different needs (e.g., health, educational, and logistical). Patients also want to feel comfortable, see the provider's office, meet the provider, and "kind of kick the tires, so to speak," a MTF explained, to know that they will be cared for. However, that is not always possible especially when patients live far away. To meet those needs, some MTFs offered video tours of clinics or video/phone calls with the providers. In one situation the MTF introduced a five-star rating system, like is found on travel websites, that provided information on the clinic and allowed former patients to rate their experience.

Aside from working with the patients, the companies also advised their Mexican medical provider partners on how to advertise, set up their offices, and how to offer the type of care that U.S. residents want. This frequently entailed an employee of the MTF company visiting the clinic either before they started working with the provider or when patients complained about their experience with that provider. For example, one company helped a plastic surgeon update his advertising strategy because his advertisements used women "who looked like strippers, and most women [in the U.S.] don't want to look like a stripper." In another instance, one of the companies consulted a PCP on how to decorate their office, greet their patients, and on some of the social/cultural differences between them and their patients. As a result, MTFs play a crucial role in linking patients and providers, by helping providers create and advertise the medical experience that patients want and by helping patients navigate a complex medical system through providing them with enough information to make medical decisions.

Mexican Medical Providers

Mexican medical providers are keenly aware of the complaints that their patients had of the U.S. healthcare system and the concerns that patients had about the quality of care that they provided in Mexico. In the interviews, many patients asked, "Is Mexico safe?" "Do the doctors have the know-how to properly treat a patient?" and "Will I get the kind of care that I want?" Their concerns were often amplified in spectacular media accounts of U.S.

patients who suffered from medical complications in Mexico or through stories that are shared among border residents that often take on the qualities of urban myths. Moreover, concerns about quality and the potential dangers of traveling abroad for care are not just stories, but are real problems cited by the Centers for Disease Control and Protection (2017). Still, the very reason why patients are willing to use Mexican healthcare is because it is different and sometimes less expensive than what they have access to in the United States. This often puts Mexican medical providers in a precarious position where they must be both different from the U.S. healthcare system, but similar enough to assuage patient concerns over safety and quality.

"Anything along the border is a conglomeration of Mexican and American thinking," including healthcare, a Texas pediatrician explained to me. "How do you compete for patients? Make them happy!" he continued, and "that is what Mexican doctors do." In practice this meant that Mexican medical providers advertised, "U.S. Trained," "English Spoken," or "Modern Technology" to link themselves to the technological and training aspect of the U.S. healthcare system that many patients are accustomed to and assume to be benchmarks of quality care. Then to distinguish themselves from U.S. healthcare, they focused on the emotional aspects of the medical encounter though spending more time with patients, developing relationships (especially with primary care), emphasizing shared decision-making, and trying to remove barriers to access (e.g., insurance, cost, and navigation) which helped put patients at ease.

For instance, Dr. Maria's office is located just a few blocks from one of the main border crossings. She moved there several years before so that it would be more convenient for her patients and because she can make more money seeing U.S. patients. Walking into her office is just like any other in the United States, with the waiting room decorated with watercolor paintings, copies of *US Weekly* and *Time* magazine on the table, and a television on mute playing cable news (usually CNN). However, there is no receptionist and Dr. Maria greets everyone personally when they walk in the door. Patients never wait more than a couple of minutes to see her and the waiting room is more for family and friends of the patient than for the patient themselves. Patient visits last as "long as they need to" she explained and if she has another patient waiting and she has to end the visit, she will call or visit the patient at their home (for those who live close by in Texas) if they have any questions. Moreover, all her patients have her personal cell phone number and can call her whenever they need to although, she discourages them from calling after eight at night.

Concerns over patient confidentially are also more relaxed, making the entire experience feel more personal. There is a guest book with several hundred entries in the waiting room where patients can sign their name, hometown/country, and leave a message for the next patient. Dr. Maria focuses on building and developing relationships not only between herself and patients, but between patients themselves, as part of her patient care approach. Reflecting, she explained that patients can be nervous or scared and that they want someone to talk to and provide them guidance. In short, they want a personal relationship with their medical provider. Moreover, she believes that it is impossible to diagnosis someone without talking to them first and getting to know them and their families. The type of experience that she provides and what her patients often commented on, was the personal aspects, particularly the relationship that they developed with her. In discussing the experience of seeing her, patients also mentioned that it was easy to get an appointment, she respected their time, and that they knew what everything was going to cost since she did not take insurance.

Dr. Maria explained that patients came to her because of her location, lower cost, and for the personalized care experience that she offers. Moreover, she explained that these experiences also put patients at ease and assured them that the type of care that they received in Mexico was indeed good. In many cases the best advertising was from her patients, she continued, who told their friends and family members and encouraged them to see her.

While it might seem that the type of care that Dr. Maria, and other Mexican doctors provided is very similar to what is in the United States, all the Mexican medical providers interviewed explained how the care that they provide is different and what patients *really* want. For instance, one surgeon explained, "many doctors [in the U.S.] just want to make a lot of money and that is unethical and if they really worried about the patients then they should charge less," suggesting that they [Mexican providers] care more about patients. A primary care provider further expanded how they are different, "people come because of the cost, it is cheaper, they get better treatment, and they have more confidence." While juxtaposing the cost difference and emphasizing how financing undermines the caring relationship was mentioned frequently, some providers also discussed how treatment and caring is approached differently in Mexico.

> U.S. doctors will treat the pain, order treatments, prescribe medications etc. without knowing the cause, I do not do that. I spend time with the patient, work slowly, ask questions and learn that maybe the pain, headache, is caused by lack of sleep, poor eating . . . I treat them like a human.

The idea that the care they provide is more "human" or "personal" was mentioned in several provider interviews and by the patients they treated and was often contrasted to the dehumanizing practices of the U.S. healthcare system. To provide that human, personal care meant to them that they talked with their patients, got to know them, understood them to be a unique person, and promoted share-decision-making, all central aspects of PPC. It also included making the experience as comfortable for the patient as possible, as in the cases of the dentist who installed massaging chairs to relax nervous patients, or the surgeon who helped arrange a patient's travel or the primary care provider who sent an employee to the pharmacy to refill a patient's prescription.

DISCUSSION

Almost 20 years after the Institute of Medicine recommended that PCC be incorporated into all medical encounters and 10 years after the ACA created incentives for medical providers to improve the patient experience, limited progress has been made. Research from all across the United States has shown that during the clinical encounter patients continue to feel that they are not being cared for and that PCC strategies are not being utilized (see Mulligan and Castenda 2017; Dalstrom 2020). Furthermore, patients often complain that the system is expensive, confusing, and that they have difficulties making medical decisions, all of which limit access to medical care, and result in negative perceptions of the U.S. healthcare system. Consequently, many individuals travel to Mexico for a wide array of medical services ranging from primary care to complex surgeries. These journeys, both big and small, illustrate both the challenges of accessing affordable, quality care in the United States and the type for medical experience that patients desire in Mexico. Furthermore, it shows how medical providers and medical travel facilitators work together to provide the type of medical encounter that patients want and how that model can be applied to the way that care is provided in the United States.

The work of Kangas (2007), has shown that medical travel can be a response to the poor quality of local health systems and the possibility of obtaining better care abroad. Care though, can have many meanings for medical travelers. For those leaving healthcare systems that are underfund, have limited resources, and/or poor outcomes, better care could mean simply access to medical care is not available locally. However, for those who travel from countries or locations that can provide the medical services needed, the type of care that a patient wants can be more nuanced accounting for both the ability to access the service and the way that the healthcare is delivered. As MTFs explained to me, Americans want to get better and expect that "the experience is personal," incorporates aspects of "customer service," and that "they will be cared for." Some researchers have characterized this model of care that medical travelers want as world class, high-tech, and/or familiar

(Sobo, Herlihy, and Bicker 2011; Milstein and Smith 2006) highlighting both the technical and cultural aspects of the experience. However, in her work on Americans who travel to Europe for IVF, Speier (2016) noted that patients want more than just low-cost, high-tech treatment, they want personal, attentive care, that includes empathy and emotional comfort. This notion of what care should consist of is similar to Kleinman's (2007) understanding of good care which includes "acknowledgement, concern, affirmation, assistance, responsibility, solidarity, and all the emotional and practical acts that enable life." (7) It also extends to all aspects of living with and/or curing a disease or ailment. In this respect, the act of providing good care is not transactional and does not have a set beginning or end, but is an open-ended process of improving the patient's situation (Mol 2008). It is also individualized, personal, and addresses a patient's physical and emotional needs along with facilitating access to the treatment needed. Yet, this type of care is not often provided within the U.S. healthcare system. In part this is the result of the emphasis on individual choice and responsibility within healthcare that has disrupted long standing notions of care and with it the patient-provider relationship (Mol 2008). It is also linked to the high cost of medical care, cost control mechanisms, the healthcare bureaucracy, and insurance coverage (or lack thereof) that further limit the time that providers can spend in the United States (Mulligan and Castañeda 2017).

To understand how current care practices do not meet patients' needs and how to potentially improve them, it is instructive to explore both the reasons why American engage in medical travel and what are their expectations for the type of care they receive in Mexico. Medical travelers often talk about their experience seeking care abroad through comparing it to medical care in the United States (Ackerman 2010; Dalstrom 2013). Often these narratives include detailed descriptions of how the system failed them in terms of costs, difficulty finding a provider, and insurance barriers. Many also mentioned that the visit was short, that their questions were not answered, and that their provider just wanted to rush them out. This made it difficult for patients to develop relationships with their providers and undermined their ability to make medical decisions (such as picking a treatment strategy), manage their chronic conditions, and/or coordinating their care with other providers. While most of these critiques are the consequences of how the health care system is organized, and not indicative of how U.S. medical providers feel, their actions were often interpreted as impersonal, cold, and profit focused, which has been reported in other medical travel research (Ackerman 2010; Speier 2016).

These perceptions were then juxtaposed to a "more caring," and personal medical encounter in Mexico where the provider spent more time, was empathetic, and was attentive to the "experience of care," by making it feel similar to home through office aesthetics and the use of English. In some situations, where a patient used a full service MTF, making medical decisions, planning the trip, arranging the transfer of medical records, and in selecting a medical provider were discussed as "easier than the U.S.," they "were helpful," and that it "helped put me at ease." Moreover, both Mexican medical providers and MTFs emphasized the necessity of providing patients with the information and guidance needed to make medical decisions and navigate the healthcare system. However, the decision to offer this type of care experience, which transcend just the clinical encounter occurred, not necessarily because Mexican medical providers and MTF are more altruistic or concerned about the patient experience, but because in many cases they have to overcome patients' logistic barriers and concerns about treatment.

Often traveling to Mexico for healthcare, even for primary care, can be logistically challenging for those who live close to the U.S./Mexico border. It is even more difficult for patients who live far away, have limited knowledge of Mexico, and are sick as in the case of Sharron, who was discussed at the beginning of this chapter. To help patients overcome these barriers and plan their trip, MTFs provide a type of medical hospitality (Cormany and Baloglu 2011), that includes trip planning, attention to the experience of the journey, the provision of information about the procedure, and patient reviews. In some situations they also help patients navigate the health system, arrange medical appointments, and transfer medical records, essentially blending the roles of a nurse navigator and a travel agent.

In addition to the logistic challenges of accessing care abroad, many U.S. residents are also apprehensive about the quality of care provided in Mexico. Therefore, as Hoffman, Crooks, and Snyder (2018), have noted, Mexican medical providers are often held at a higher standard than their U.S. counterparts and the way that they provide care is often based on their need to validate their medical knowledge. Thus, they have to offer a care experience that this perceived as better than what patients receive in the United States. This is often accomplished though clinic aesthetics, that create a sense of familiarity, working with MTFs to make access easier, and by providing emphatic care, which has also been documented in medical journeys to India and Costa Rica (Solomon 2011; Ackerman 2010). It also engages patients by guiding them through their care trajectory instead of expecting them to take full responsibility.

Numerous researchers have highlighted the importance of affective labor and how it comforts patients and supports the development of emotional connections between medical providers and patients (Vindrola-Padros 2020; Ackerman 2010). According to Speier (2016) the affective labor and discourse used by medical providers and MTFs are central to the care experience, "colors patients perceptions . . . [and is] interpreted as altruism (65). The importance implementing these approaches into patients healthcare trajectory is that it not only helps overcome some of their concerns about traveling and the quality of care abroad, but it improves their overall perception of the care received. This approach is so effective that when implemented appropriately, patients also have the propensity to overly romanticize the level of care that they are provided (Inhorn and Patrizo 2015; Solomon 2011) and become "brand ambassadors" for the medical provider (Ackerman 2010).

This illustrates that many medical travelers are looking for more than just a provider who can do a procedure in Mexico, they wanted to be assured that the care experience was better than the United States. For many participants that did not mean that they were given more choices, but that they were helped throughout the entire medical encounter, treated like an individual, and that their emotional needs were addressed. Moreover, it meant that the responsibility of navigating the healthcare system and in making medical decisions was not theirs alone, but shared with medical providers and MTFs. Thus, through providing empathetic care (not more choices) at all stages of the medical encounter and attending to the logistic challenges of accessing medical care, Mexican medical providers were able to overcome patients' negative perceptions of Mexico, the logistic barriers of accessing care, and provide a type of care that Americans preferred.

TOWARD A NEW MODEL OF HEALTH IN THE UNITED STATES

Even though integrating PCC into U.S. medical practices has been difficult, the passage of the ACA has created space where certain U.S. medical providers can incorporate the PCC strategies used by Mexican providers and MTFs into the type of care that they offer. The ACA requires almost all adults earning over 138 percent of the Federal Poverty Line to be insured either through their employer or through the health insurance exchanges. This requirement has unintentionally contributed to the growth of two models of care that operate similarly to Mexican medical providers and could be further improved by applying lessons learned from studying medical travel more broadly. The first is direct primary care also referred to as concierge medicine. Direct primary care is where patients pay a one-time (or annual) registration fee, and a monthly fee directly to a primary care provider (PCP). Then enrolled patients get unlimited same day visits for non-emergency cases, more time with their primary care provider, do not have to get insurance approval for care provided by their PCP, and providers claim that they can offer more personalized care (Luthia 2016). This is because under the ACA, patients enrolled in direct primary care are exempt from purchasing a comprehensive health insurance plan and only need catastrophic coverage which is significantly less expensive than the cost of comprehensive health insurance. These health insurance plans generally do not cover primary care so it also decouples the provider from much of the insurance billing reducing some of their operating costs and allows providers more flexibility in how they deliver and market the caring experience.

For secondary and tertiary care, the ACA's requirement that many employers provide health insurance has led to the growth of self-funded insurance plans. Under these plans, the employer assumes all the finical risk and, therefore, is incentivized to find lower cost healthcare for their employees. In some situations, this has resulted in them encouraging their employees to get surgeries and medical care at hospitals (sometimes in other states) that provide care at lower costs (Carbello 2013). To compete for these patient hospitals such as Kalispell Regional Hospital in Montana have developed a medical travel program staffed with medical concierge nurses who receive training from the Medical Tourism Association, a medical travel trade group. Using the MTF model, the program focuses on the patient-centered aspects of care such as personal relationships, price transparency through bundled payments, hospitality, and patient navigation. In addition, the nurses work with the patients throughout the entire process from first contact to after the surgery through blending traditional elements of care coordination (e.g., arranging medical appointments, transferring medical records and postoperative care) with hospitality (e.g., referrals to hotels). These types of programs are in their infancy and are not widely available, nevertheless they demonstrate that the type of care strategies used in medical travel can be applied to domestic healthcare. They also highlight that what patients want, and what makes them engaged in their healthcare is not giving them more choices, but providing with them with more care and support.

Both of these models have gained popularity in the United States because of systemic problems with how healthcare is delivered. They are also areas when medical providers have more latitude in how they deliver care and could make significant changes. Understanding why a patient would travel to Mexico for care, the type of care they want, and how that care is provided is instructive for thinking about how these two models could be strengthened and expanded to other patients. Research on medical travel to Mexico suggests that many patients want a different care giving experience, one that expands beyond the clinical encounter. It also underscores, how personalizing medical care, incorporating empathy, and caring (in the expansive sense of the word), can assuage patient concerns and is the type of healthcare experience that many patients want. As the amount of doctors who want to start practicing direct primary/concierge medicine grow along with amount of health systems who want to attract patients from outside their traditional service area, it is important to understand how MTFs and Mexican medical providers work together to provide a type of medical care that is more personal, less bureaucratic, and hopefully more affordable for patients.

REFERENCES

Aboumatar, Hanan J., Bickey, H. Chang, Jad Al Danaf, Mohammad Shaear, Ruth Namuyinga, Sathyanarayanan Elumalai, Jill A. Marsteller, and Peter J. Pronovost. 2015. "Promising Practices for Achieving Patient-Centered Hospital Care." *Medical Care* 53(9): 758–767.

Ackerman, Sara L. 2010. "Plastic Paradise: Transforming Bodies and Selves in Costa Rica's Cosmetic Surgery Tourism Industry." *Medical Anthropology* 29(4): 403–423.

Adams, Krystyna, Jeremy Snyder, Valorie A. Crooks, and Nicole S. Berry. 2017. "Stay Cool, Sell Stuff Cheap, and Smile: Examining How Reputational Management of Dental Tourism Reinforces Structural Oppression in Los Algodones, Mexico." *Social Science & Medicine* 190: 157–164.

Balint, Michael. 1955. "The Doctor, His Patient, and the Illness." *The Lancet* 265(6866): 683–688.

Bergmark, Regan, Donald Barr, and Ronald Garcia. 2010. "Mexican Immigrants in the US Living Far from the Border may Return to Mexico for Health Services." *Journal of Immigrant and Minority Health* 12(4): 610–614.

Berry, Judith A. 2009. "Nurse Practitioner/Patient Communication Styles in Clinical Practice." *The Journal for Nurse Practitioners* 5(7): 508–515.

Carabello, Laura. 2013. "US Domestic Medical Tourism Delivers Sustainable Tourism for America's Cities and States." *Journal of Tourism and Hospitality* 2(2): 1–3.

Centers for Disease Control and Prevention. 2017. "Medical Tourism." Accessed January 1, 2020. https://wwwnc.cdc.gov/travel/page/medical-tourism

Chee, Heng Leng, Andrea Whittaker, and Heong Hong Por. 2017. "Medical Travel Facilitators, Private Hospitals and International Medical Travel in Assemblage." *Asia Pacific Viewpoint* 58(2): 242–254.

Committee on Quality of Health Care in America, and Institute of Medicine Staff. 2001.
Crossing the Quality Chasm: A New Health System for the 21st Century. Accessed December 12, 2019. https://www.ncbi.nlm.nih.gov/books/NBK222274/

Cormany, Dan, and Seyhmus Baloglu. 2011. "Medical Travel Facilitator Websites: An Exploratory Study of Web Page Contents and Services Offered to the Prospective Medical Tourist." *Tourism Management* 32(4): 709–716.

Crooks, Valorie A., Neville Li, Jeremy Snyder, Shafik Dharamsi, Shelly Benjaminy, Karen J. Jacob, and Judy Illness. 2015. "You Don't Want to Lose that Trust that You've Built with this Patient": (Dis)Trust, Medical Tourism, and the Canadian Family Physician-Patient Relationship." *BMC Family Practice* 16: 25–25.

Dalen, James E., and Joseph S. Alpert. 2019. "Medical Tourists: Incoming and Outgoing." *The American Journal of Medicine* 132(1): 9–10.

Dalstrom, Matthew. 2013. "Medical Travel Facilitators: Connecting Patients and Providers in a Globalized World." *Anthropology & Medicine* 20(1): 24–35.

Dalstrom Matthew. 2020. "Medicaid, Motherhood, and the Challenges of Having a Healthy Pregnancy Amidst Changing Social Networks." *Women Birth* 33(3): e302–e308.

Dalstrom, Matthew, Ryan Chung, and Lynette Castronovo. 2020. "Impacting Health through Cross-Border Pharmaceutical Purchases." *Medical Anthropology* 39(2): 182–195.

Da Silva, Chantal. 2019. "Thousands of Americans are Crossing the Border into Mexico Every Year to Get Affordable Medical Treatment." *Newsweek* Accessed February 12, 2020. https://www.newsweek.com/thousands-americans-cross-border-mexico-affordable-medical-treatment-each-1426943

Dwamena, F., Holmes-Rovner, M., Gaulden, C. M., Jorgenson, S., Sadigh, G., Sikorskii, A., Lewin, S., Smith, R. C., Coffey, J., Olomu, A., and Beasley, M. 2012. "Interventions for Providers to Promote a Patient-Centered Approach in Clinical Consultations." *Cochrane Database of Systematic Reviews* 12: CD003267.

Finefrock, Doug, Sridhar Patel, David Zodda, Themba Nyirenda, Richard Nierenberg, Joseph Feldman, and Chinwe Ogedegbe. 2018 "Patient-Centered Communication Behaviors that Correlate with Higher Patient Satisfaction Scores." *Journal of Patient Experience* 5(3): 231–235.

Gerteis, Margaret, Susan Edgman-Levitan, Jennifer Daley, and Thomas L. Delbanco, eds. 1993. *Through the Patient's Eyes: Understanding And Promoting Patient-Centered Care*. Jossey-Bass.

Hashim, M. Jawad. 2017, "Patient-Centered Communication: Basic Skills." *American Family Physician* 95(1): 29–34.

Hoffman, Leon, Jeremy Snyder, and Valorie Crooks. 2018. "A Challenging Entanglement: Health Care providers' Perspectives on Caring for Ill and Injured Tourists on Cozumel Island, Mexico." *International Journal of Qualitative Studies on Health and Well-Being* 13(1): 1479583.

Horton, Sarah, and Stephanie Cole. 2011. "Medical Returns: Seeking Health Care in Mexico." *Social Science & Medicine* 72(11): 1846–1852.

Inhorn, Marcia. 2018. *Cosmopolitan Conceptions: IVF Sojourns in Global Dubai*. Duke University Press.

Inhorn, Marcia C., and Pasquale Patrizio. 2015. "Infertility Around the Globe: New Thinking on Gender, Reproductive Technologies and Global Movements in the 21st Century." *Human Reproduction Update* 21(4): 411–426.

Johnston, Rory, Valorie A. Crooks, Krystyna Adams, Jeremy Snyder, and Paul Kingsbury. 2011. "An Industry Perspective on Canadian Patients' Involvement in Medical Tourism: Implications for Public Health." *BMC Public Health* 11: 416–416.

Kaiser Family Foundation. 2019. Health Costs. Accessed December 12, 2019. https://www.kff.org/health-costs/

Kangas, Beth. 2002. "Therapeutic Itineraries in a Global World: Yemenis and Their Search for Biomedical Treatment Abroad." *Medical Anthropology* 21(1): 35–78.

Kangas, Beth. 2007. "Hope from Abroad in the International Medical Travel of Yemeni Patients." *Anthropology & Medicine* 14(3): 293–305.

Kiwanuka, Frank, Shah Jahan Shayan, and Agbele Alaba Tolulope. 2019. "Barriers to Patient and Family-Centered Care in Adult Intensive Care Units: A Systematic Review." *Nursing Open* 6(3): 676–684.

Kleinman, A. 2007. "Today's Biomedicine and Caregiving: Are They Incompatible to the Point of Divorce?" University of Leiden: Cleveringa Lecture, Nov. 26.

Laine, Christine, and Frank Davidoff. 1996. "Patient-Centered Medicine: A Professional Evolution." *JAMA* 275(2): 152–156.

Lunt, Neil, Daniel Horsfall, and Johanna Hanefeld. 2016. "Medical Tourism: A Snapshot of Evidence on Treatment Abroad." *Maturitas* 88: 37–44.

Luthia. 2016. "Fueled By Health Law, 'Concierge Medicine' Reaches New Markets." Kaiser Family Foundation. Accessed November 12, 2019. https://khn.org/news/fueled-by-health-law-concierge-medicine-reaches-new-markets/

Mason, A. 2014. "Overcoming the 'Dual-Delivery' Stigma: A Review of Patient-Centeredness in the Costa Rica Medical Tourism Industry." *The International Journal of Communication and Health* 4: 1–9.

McCullough, Kimberly and Matthew Dalstrom. 2018. "I Am Insured But How Do I Use My Coverage: Lessons from the Front Lines of Medicaid Reform." *Public Health Nursing* 35(6): 568–573.

McKinney, Maureen. 2011. "About that Quality Chasm: 10 Years After IOM Report, Authors See Progress, But…". Accessed October 10, 2019. https://www.modernhealthcare.com/article/20110221/MAGAZINE/110219950/about-that-quality-chasm

Millenson, M.L and J. Marci. 2012. "Will the Affordable Care Act Move Patient-Centeredness to Center Stage?" Urban Institute. Accessed November 10, 2019. http://www.urban.org/sites/default/files/alfresco/publication-pdfs/412524-Will-the-Affordable-Care-ActMove-Patient-Centeredness-to-Center-Stage-.PDF

Milstein, Arnold, and Mark Smith. 2006. "America's New Refugees—Seeking Affordable Surgery Offshore." *New England Journal of Medicine* 355(16): 1637–1640.

Moerman, Daniel E. 2002. *Meaning, Medicine, and the" Placebo Effect"*. Cambridge University Press.

Mol, Annemarie. 2008. *The Logic of Care: Health and the Problem of Patient Choice*. Routledge.

Mulligan, Jessica. 2017. "The Problem of Choice: From the Voluntary Way to Affordable Care Act Health Insurance Exchanges." *Social Science & Medicine* 181: 34–42.

Mulligan, Jessica M., and Heide Castañeda, eds. 2017. *Unequal Coverage: The Experience of Health Care Reform in the United States*. NYU Press.

Oberle, Alex P., and Daniel D. Arreola. 2004. "Mexican Medical Border Towns: A Case Study of Algodones, Baja California." *Journal of Borderlands Studies* 19(2): 27–44.

Ormond, Meghann and Matthew Sothern. 2012. "You, Too, Can Be an International Medical Traveler: Reading Medical Travel Guidebooks." *Health & Place* 18(5): 935–941.

Politi, Mary C., Kimberly A. Kaphingst, Matthew Kreuter, Enbal Shacham, Melissa C. Lovell, and Timothy McBride. 2014. "Knowledge of Health Insurance

Terminology and Details Among the Uninsured." *Medical Care Research and Review* 71(1): 85–98.

Premji Kamila, Ross Upshur, France Légaré, and Kevein Pottie. 2014. "Future of Family Medicine: Role of Patient-Centred Care and Evidence-Based Medicine." *Canadian Family Physician* 60(5): 409–412.

Rylko-Bauer, Barbara and Paul Farmer. 2002. "Managed Care or Managed Inequality? A Call for Critiques of Market-Based Medicine." *Medical Anthropology Quarterly* 16(4): 476–502.

Sered, Susan. 2018. "Uninsured in America: Before and After the ACA." In *Unequal Coverage The Experience of Health Care Reform in the United States*, edited by Heidi Castañeda and Jessica Mulligan, 156–176. New York: New York University Press.

Snyder, Jeremy, Valorie A. Crooks, Krystyna Adams, Paul Kingsbury, and Rory Johnston. 2011. "The 'Patient's Physician One-Step Removed': The Evolving Roles of Medical Tourism Facilitators." *Journal of Medical Ethics* 37(9): 530–534.

Sobo, Elisa J. 2009. "Medical Travel: What it Means, Why it Matters." *Medical Anthropology* 28(4): 326–335.

Sobo, Elisa J., Elizabeth Herlihy, and Mary Bicker. 2011. "Selling Medical Travel to US Patient-Consumers: The Cultural Appeal of Website Marketing Messages." *Anthropology and Medicine* 18(1): 119–136.

Solomon, Harris. 2011. "Affective Journeys: The Emotional Structuring of Medical Tourism in India." *Anthropology & Medicine* 18(1): 105–118.

Speier, Amy. 2016. *Fertility Holidays: IVF Tourism and the Reproduction of Whiteness*. New York University Press.

Su, Dejun, Chad Richardson, Ming Wen, and José A. Pagán. 2011. "Cross-Border Utilization of Health Care: Evidence from a Population-Based Study in South Texas." *Health Services Research* 46(3): 859–876.

Victoor, Aafke, Diana MJ Delnoij, Roland D. Friele, and Jany Rademakers. 2012. "Determinants of Patient Choice of Healthcare Providers: A Scoping Review." *BMC Health Services Research* 12(1): 272.

Vindrola-Padros, Cecilia. 2019. *Critical Ethnographic Perspectives on Medical Travel*. Routledge.

Wolf, Debra M., Lisa Lehman, Robert Quinlin, Thomas Zullo, and Leslie Hoffman. 2008. "Effect of Patient-Centered Care on Patient Satisfaction and Quality of Care." *Journal of Nursing Care Quality* 23(4): 316–321.

Chapter 5

"Caring for" and "Caring about" International Patients in Delhi

Medical Travel Facilitation between Strategy and Sympathy

Sarah Hartmann

In a hospital in central Delhi, India, two Omani patients, a man in his twenties and a slightly older man, arrive at the main entrance. With a big smile on his face, Tariq,[1] an Indian medical travel facilitator, approaches them, says hello and shakes hands. He asks: "How are you? How was the flight? How is Oman?" The younger man, Kamal, says that he is doing well, points thumbs up for the flight and notes that it is not as cold in Oman as it is in Delhi right now. "I told you!" replies Tariq, laughs and slaps him affably on the back. He knows Kamal already as he facilitated his medical treatment a few months ago. Kamal has returned to Delhi for a follow-up check. In addition, he has brought his uncle along who is suffering from undiagnosed back pain and asks Tariq whether he or his uncle is going to see the doctor first. Tariq says that it depends on the doctors' availability. Tariq guides his patients through the maze-like corridors; he walks ahead towards the north wing of the hospital, and the patients follow faithfully.

(From field notes, Delhi 2015, names changed)

The situation described here is typical and extraordinary at the same time; typical because on a regular basis hundreds of international medical travelers arrive in private hospitals in Delhi National Capital Region (NCR), which includes the metropolitan area of Delhi and surrounding cities, a notable and well-established destination on the transnational healthcare market, maybe not so well-known in Western countries but definitely at a high rate for patients coming from neighboring countries, the Middle East, countries in central Asia and different African countries (FICCI 2017). Extraordinary is the situation because submitting oneself to medical treatment abroad, in an unfamiliar city far from home presents an extraordinary challenge for most international patients. Decisions need to be taken that affect one's health severely, for better or worse, ranging from finding a reliable doctor and selecting the right treatment option to coping with practical and emotional distress in the unfamiliar environment. This is where an economic actor comes forward to make available a remedy: medical travel facilitators—like Tariq in the scene described in the field notes above—offer assistance to international patients throughout their medical travel endeavor and connect them to healthcare providers abroad.

International medical travel, or medical value travel as some industry players like to call it (FICCI 2017, p. 16), has undergone major shifts over the last decades in terms of the actors involved (e.g., healthcare and other service providers, insurance companies, policy makers etc.), the healthcare arrangements on offer, the number of patients becoming medical travelers and its geographic scope (see, e.g., Ormond & Lunt 2019; Connell 2015; Casey et al. 2013; Ormond 2013). While much has been written about the general configuration of transnational healthcare markets, destination marketing, patients' reasons to travel abroad, and their experiences (Connell 2015; Bell et al. 2015; Whittaker 2015; Kingsbury et al. 2012; Crooks et al. 2010), less is known about the work practices of intermediaries that are known by different names, for example, medical travel agents, healthcare facilitators, case managers or patient navigators. Although medical travel facilitators are considered to "play a substantial and evolving role in the practice of medical tourism" (Snyder et al. 2011, p. 530) and are described as "crucial connectors between foreign patients and host countries" (Wagle 2013, p. 28), the work they do in terms of providing support at the destination site and especially their contribution to the care provided to international patients have gained little attention in academic literature so far (but see for example Dalstrom 2013; Hartmann 2017).

Based on an ethnographic case study conducted in Delhi NCR in 2015, this chapter aims to shed light on the practices of medical travel facilitators who are based at a medical travel destination site in the Global South. It will illustrate that the medical travel facilitation model practiced in Delhi consists in a comprehensive and individualized support of international patients whereby facilitators engage in a broad range of tasks. Drawing on the empirical findings, I suggest that many of the practices performed by these facilitators can actually be conceptualized as care work. To support this argument, the chapter firstly explains in what ways medical travel facilitation comprises care work. To do so, it mainly draws upon care work as theorized by Lynch and McLaughlin (1995) who differentiate between different dimensions of care and especially between "caring *for*" and "caring *about*." This conceptual approach offers a fresh look at the range of practices performed in medical travel facilitation and the underlying rationales. This raises questions about how caring relations are negotiated in a commercial context. Secondly, this chapter illuminates some of the intricacies of the setting in which such care work is performed, unraveling seemingly contradicting rationales of sympathy and business strategy. This contribution then challenges the theoretical dichotomy between social and economic rationales, which does not necessarily apply to the realities on the ground.

TRANSNATIONAL HEALTHCARE AND MEDICAL TRAVEL TO DELHI

While patients seeking healthcare abroad is not a new phenomenon, over the past decades international medical travel has become a rapidly evolving industry. Patients travel across national boundaries to receive healthcare services at destinations tailored to serve the needs of international customers (Kaspar & Reddy 2017; Botterill et al. 2013; Mainil et al. 2012; Whittaker et al. 2010). In the context of globalization, neoliberal restructuring of healthcare sectors and its integration into supranational bodies has changed the healthcare landscape. In the mid-1990s, the World Trade Organisation (WTO) issued the General Agreement on Trade in Services Act that liberalized international trade in health and defined the "Movement of Consumers" as one of four modes of healthcare supply (Blouin et al. 2006, p. 210). Such regulations set in a global arena and market-based competition has resulted in shifts in terms of medical travel destination locations (Connell 2013; Herrick 2007). Since the late twentieth century, countries of the Global South and particularly Asian countries such as India have positioned themselves successfully as destinations in the global healthcare market (Connell 2013; Reddy & Qadeer 2010; Connell 2006).

Following restructuring of the healthcare sector in the 1990s that led to privatization (Reddy & Qadeer 2010, p. 70), India was able to establish itself as one of the leading medical travel destinations in Asia. Indian healthcare providers promote advanced technology, state of the art infrastructure, relative cost advantages, and doctors with proficiency in several medical disciplines (Lunt & Mannion 2014; Smith 2012; Reddy & Qadeer 2010; Herrick 2007; Connell 2006). Delhi NCR is a known healthcare hub in India (Sen Gupta 2015, p. 230; Dawn & Pal 2011, p. 2; Hazarika 2010). Several corporate hospital chains are present there that have a considerable share of international patients ranging up to 50 percent in certain cases (Kaspar & Reddy 2017, p. 231). According to the informants participating in this study most of the international patients that come to Delhi are from the Middle East, from South Asian Association for Regional Cooperation countries (SAARC), countries of the Commonwealth of Independent States (CIS), and different African countries. This prevalent mobility pattern positions this case study in a South–South medical travel context, which is said to make the biggest share of medical travel (Ormond & Sulianti 2014; Connell 2011) despite many studies and media coverage in Europe often focusing on North-South medical travel.

CONCEPTUALIZING CARE WORK IN MEDICAL TRAVEL

In the introduction of a special issue published on transnational healthcare, Bell et al. (2015, p. 288) call attention to the "under-examined role and dimensions of formal and informal care work involved in international medical travel." This book is thus a great opportunity to explore different dimensions and layers of care in this particular context and this chapter contributes by conceptualizing some aspects of medical travel facilitation as care work and discussing the implications thereof. Up to now, care and care work have been related to medical travel facilitation only relatively loosely. Based on the study of Casey et al. (2013) that ascribes the attendants of international patients three roles, namely the one of a knowledge broker, a navigator and a companion, Ormond et al. (2014) argue that medical travel facilitators can take on these roles as well. Elaborating on the role of a companion, they suggests that facilitators "may engage in formal emotional labour to provide medical travellers with companionship and support" (Ormond et al. 2014, p. 12). Similarly, Whittaker and Speier (2010, p. 363) address affective labor involved in the work of medical travel facilitators in the context of cross-border reproductive travel. The authors find that "companies such as these [medical facilitation company] reinsert the discourse of affective labor, care, and nurturing within a reproductive experience that is otherwise devoid of all familiar relationships" (Whittaker & Speier 2010, p. 372).

In the following, care work is introduced as a conceptual route into better understanding the work practiced by medical travel facilitators in Delhi. Care work is in itself a complex concept and has been approached by looking at different conceptualizations, purposes and dimensions, logics or issues. England and Folbre (1999, p. 40), for example, say that "caring work includes any occupation in which the worker provides a service to someone with whom he or she is in personal contact. The work is called 'caring' on the assumption that the worker responds to a need or desire that is directly expressed by the recipient." Lynch and Walsh (2009) provide a practice-oriented approach toward care work by enlisting different dimensions of care work which are particularly interesting for this contribution here. The authors say: "Care work generally involves not only *emotional work* and *moral commitment*, but also *mental work* (including a considerable amount of planning), *physical work* (doing practical tasks including body work such as lifting, touching and massaging) and *cognitive work* (using the skills of knowing how to care)" (Lynch & Walsh 2009, p. 42, italics in original). These five dimensions show that a versatile assemblage of tasks that demand the involvement of the caregiver's body, mind, and emotions constitutes care work. The authors complement these dimensions by enlisting some additional features that shape the practices of care work such as commitment and responsibility, trust, attentiveness or emotional engagement (Lynch & Walsh 2009, p. 43).

The conceptual distinction between "caring *for*" and "caring *about*" is seen as particularly insightful when thinking through care in the commodified arrangements of medical travel facilitation. Thereby, caring *for* refers to the practice of "catering for the material and other general well-being of the one receiving care" (Lynch & McLaughlin 1995, p. 256). By contrast, caring *about* refers to emotional aspects of caring and is described by Lynch and McLaughlin (1995, pp. 256–257) as "having affection and concern for the other and working on the relationship between the self and the other to ensure the development of the bond." This distinction is relevant, as these forms of care work involve varying qualities and different practices. Prompted by the question about the ability to commodify care work, the authors question "the extent to which 'caring about' itself can be developed within commodified 'caring for' relations" (Lynch & McLaughlin 1995, p. 257). This goes hand in hand with "the question about the divisibility of 'caring for' and 'caring about'" (Lynch & McLaughlin 1995, p. 257). The authors argue that sometimes they cannot be easily divided since caring *about* may be expressed though practicing caring *for* and in return caring *for* "may yet permit the development of 'caring about' at least sometimes and to some extent" (Lynch & McLaughlin 1995, p. 275). It is the latter case that this contribution is going to exemplify and elaborate.

Issues around the emotional dimension and commodification of care work, its facets and implications have also been discussed elsewhere in the rich body of academic literature on care and care work (Hochschild 1983; England & Folbre 1999; Folbre & Nelson 2000; Madörin 2009; Green & Lawson 2011). A seminal contribution to this debate is Hochschild's (1979, p. 561) conceptualization of "emotion work" as "the act of trying to change in degree or quality an emotion or feeling" which can also be commodified and exchanged on the market as "emotional labour." There are extensive debates about the question if or to what extent care work can be commodified, which dimensions and tasks are commodifiable and what its commodification implies (see, e.g., Lynch & Walsh 2009; Folbre & Nelson 2000; Hochschild 2003; Madörin 2013). In the following section, the extent and motivation with which medical travel facilitators engage in emotion work of some sort will be critically analyzed and discussed in the commercial context of transnational healthcare.

A NOTE ON DATA COLLECTION AND A BRIEF INTRODUCTION OF THE PARTICIPANTS

This study is based on qualitative data collected during two months of ethnographic fieldwork in Delhi NCR. Between December 2014 and February 2015, I conducted over thirty interviews with representatives of medical travel companies and self-employed facilitators. Furthermore, field notes were taken on multiple days of job-shadowing during which different medical travel facilitators were accompanied on their work, mostly carried out in corporate hospitals in Delhi NCR. Complementing the interview transcripts with fieldnotes was an important methodological move since different dimensions of the facilitators' work could be captured and eventually brought about care as a recurring theme in the data.

Generally, the interviewees can be categorized as either director, respectively, employee of a medical travel company or self-employed facilitator. Out of the participants representing a medical travel company, almost all were Indians and most of them had gained work experiences in hospitals prior to their job in medical travel facilitation. The sizes of the companies for which they have worked at the time varied considerably—the number of employees lies between two and over forty. The number of patients served monthly varies accordingly; the spectrum ranges from three to over two hundred. From the eight self-employed facilitators who participated in this study, two were Indian, two were from Afghanistan and four were from Iraq. Those facilitators with migration background all came to Delhi for their studies and entered the medical travel facilitation business as a side job after being introduced to it by friends already working in the field or through personal experience of medical travel as a patient or attendant. They are usually well-positioned for this work in terms of their language skills and network connections to their home countries. Medical travel companies, in turn, usually target multiple countries for customer acquisition. The prevalent business model among the participants was based on commission fees paid by hospitals for the international patients they guide to their institution. The amount of such referral fees varies depending on the hospitals and the agreement they have with different facilitators and medical travel companies. This business model is problematic in terms of lack of transparency and challenges the facilitators' integrity toward the patients as financial incentives may guide the facilitators choice or suggestion of hospital rather than acting in the patients' best interest. The complex implications of this business model for the care work provided by medical travel facilitators will be analyzed in the following.

THE MEDICAL TRAVEL FACILITATION MODEL PRACTICED IN DELHI

Medical travel facilitators are generally understood as intermediary service providers who promote transnational healthcare, connect patients with healthcare providers abroad, provide information and advice, practical assistance and support in realizing medical travel (see for example Hartmann 2017; Ormond 2014; Dalstrom 2013; Mohamad et al. 2012; Snyder et al. 2012). The medical travel facilitators interviewed in this study explained that their work begins before the patient's stay in Delhi and continues once the patient has returned. Actually, even before medical travel facilitators get in touch with prospective patients, they need to build an operational set-up to facilitate medical travel successfully. This means that knowledge about the healthcare market in Delhi and the situation in patient source countries is acquired. Furthermore, connections with local healthcare and other service providers need to be established. Potential customers are approached and mobilized toward the Indian healthcare market following different strategies (Hartmann 2019). Then the patient's and attendant's transportation, accommodation and visa are organized, and a treatment plan finalized in consultation with the doctor and the chosen hospital. In the literature, the work of medical travel facilitators during this phase is described in multiple accounts (see for example Hanefeld et al. 2015; Snyder et al. 2012; Mohamad et al. 2012; Sobo et al. 2011; Gan & Frederick 2011; Crooks et al. 2011). What happens once the patient has arrived at the medical travel destination site, however, is not very well documented as many studies focusing on medical travel facilitators draw on website analysis or focus on individuals who are based in the patient sending countries. The study discussed here focused especially on the work of medical travel facilitators who assist patients at the destination site. The field-note section at the beginning of this chapter gave initial insights into such daily practices and the empirical data shows that the work of medical travel facilitators goes far beyond information transfer, counseling, and logistics brokering (see also Hartmann 2017). Instead it is suggested here that medical travel facilitation can to some extent be conceptualized as care work. In the next two sections, two particularly interesting aspects of the facilitation model practiced in Delhi are elaborated and analyzed in more depth drawing on the conceptual underpinnings of care work introduced earlier.

CARING *FOR* INTERNATIONAL PATIENTS

The medical travel facilitation model practiced in Delhi in terms of onsite patient assistance, as it presented itself during fieldwork, excels in an encompassing support that includes diverse flanking amenities around the patients' treatment. Some participants called it "concierge services," a term already coined by Mohamad et al. (2012, p. 360). It seems to be an essential part of the facilitators' work at the destination site and the interviewees stressed that they care for the overall well-being of "their" patients from the moment they land at the airport until they get on the plane home.

In the scene described in the beginning of this chapter, Tariq, an Indian medical travel facilitator welcomes two Omani patients and gets the day in the hospital started. Only the night before, Kamal and his uncle were received at the airport and brought to a guesthouse close to the hospital. In the first encounter, it seems that the medical travel facilitator wants to make Kamal and his uncle feel at ease showing welcoming body language and seizing on their previous conversations. The initial questions to break the ice mirror his focus upon his patients' well-being and their travel experience so far. With the question "How is Oman?" he immediately relates to them and expresses that he is informed about where they come from. When one of the men mentions that it is cold in Delhi, Tariq replies that he had told him in advance. He was in touch with the patients before their flight with a briefing on what to wear under the current weather conditions. Through email, Skype calls and WhatsApp chats, facilitators and patients can be constantly in touch, before, during and after the patients stay in India. Tariq's manager reflects upon the concierge service that his employees provide and explains what he expects from them when welcoming patients in Delhi with practical examples:

> When they [international patients] land here the case-manager receives them at the airport, start helping them from the first. Let me say, before you checkout the airport, it is always best you take a SIM card from here. Because here the SIM card will be activated within an hour, if you buy it outside it will take three days to activate. So, first piece of advice. The second piece of advice, please if you have warm clothes in your suitcase, take them out, it's cold outside. The third piece of advice, we are going directly to the hospital, it's going to take about 40 minutes, if you want to have a cup of coffee before you leave the airport, the coffee shop is right here, the coffee is on me. Okay? So, you start building up

that relationship. When the patient and the case-manager reach the hospital, the case-manager continues to help in each and every step.

Being in touch with the patient from the first moment, showing concern about his or her emotional and physical well-being and giving advice, even if it is just about small things like where to get a coffee or what clothes to wear, initiate a relationship and show that the facilitator cares for the patients in a comprehensive way. This goes beyond merely connecting patients and the healthcare providers by mediating their contact. As "medical concierges who accompany the patients throughout their time abroad" (Dalstrom 2013, p. 29) medical travel facilitators may engage in different practices that make the patients overall experience more pleasant.

Although these practices are often shaped by notions of service, drawing on some of the characteristic features of care work, it is suggested that some of the practices of medical travel facilitators assisting international patients at the destination site can also be conceptualized as care work. One of the essential features of caring for somebody according to Lynch and Walsh (2009, p. 43) is "identifying someone's needs for care and knowing how they can be met." The authors consider that as the "cognitive work" involved in care work. Indeed, the encompassing concierge service is justified by the interviewees' perception of international patients as being often stressed, helpless, and vulnerable given that they are physically weakened for suffering from a disease or injury and often additionally emotionally stressed and worried. Traveling abroad and being in an unfamiliar environment adds on another challenge. Limited capacity to evaluate the treatment options or choose a suitable hospital and doctor abroad and the danger of getting tricked by people pursuing unethical practices render international patients particularly vulnerable. Based on these circumstances and their perception of the care needs of international patients, facilitators articulate a market niche to which they respond with their extensive facilitation services in the example of the participants of this study in Delhi.

This facilitation service presents a quasi-endless list of tasks. It includes guidance, practically by leading patients through physical space (e.g., the labyrinth of corridors in hospitals or the winding alleys in Delhi) but also metaphorically by counseling and assisting patients in decision-making processes (e.g., choosing a hospital and doctor, where to stay or how much money is reasonable to spend). Then, facilitators try to smoothen the treatment pathways by wise coordination (e.g., doing the check-ups before the consultation with the doctor and ensuring the necessary documents are carried with them) and negotiation skills (e.g., treatment costs, time management) (see Hartmann 2017 for more details). Thus, a medical travel facilitator needs to be a person with foresight to anticipate possible struggles and concerns the patients and attendants may have in order to convey a feeling of being in good hands. They engage in "mental work," another facet of care work described by Lynch and Walsh (2009, p. 43), comprising attentiveness and "holding the persons and their interests in mind, keeping them 'present' in mental planning, and anticipating and prioritising their needs and interests" (Lynch & Walsh 2009, p. 45). In this sense of safeguarding the patients' needs and interests, medical travel facilitators also take the role of a patient advocate, a notion that has been coined in the literature before (Hanefeld et al. 2015; Ormond et al. 2014; Dalstrom 2013; Snyder et al. 2012; Sobo et al. 2011). This is needed if unnecessary treatment is imposed, the service is overcharged or worse, if something goes wrong during the medical procedure. Snyder et al. (2012, p. 2) even argue that "brokers can play an essential role in facilitating communication, providing information, and securing overall quality control by assessing the reputability and reliability of international facilities."

Another important task is translation, which is often underestimated in terms of its demands and responsibility as argued by Kaspar (2015) in the context of catering for the need of international patients. Thereby, medical travel facilitators not only translate from one language to another but also from medical jargon to phrases that lay person can understand. Helping themselves with simplifications and adjustments can be critical given the very sensitive issue of peoples' health. Apart from the language, there are likely to be other cultural issues that medical travelers and their attendants face in a place far from home. Thus, medical travel facilitators have learned that their engagement in cultural brokering renders a more comfortable medical travel experience to patients and contributes to preventing misunderstandings, affronts, and delays in the process.

The list of tasks and duties could go on and on; the interviewees themselves struggled to define what is and what is not part of their job. One of them gets to the heart of it by saying: "And all the thing we will do. Also, in the hospital, suppose that patient need fruits, need clothes, need anything. Any need in life, because the patient is a foreigner, okay? He does not know where his need is available. [. . .] So, this kind, e-v-e-r-y-t-h-i-n-g [knocks on the table] is agent's duty." The medical travel facilitators that participated in this study thus endeavored to care for their patients in an encompassing way, responding to the complex and multi-layered care needs of the international patients. Providing such a "concierge service" can be conceptualized as services flanking direct medical care, respectively, as "the other necessary activities that provide the preconditions for personal caregiving" (Razavi 2007, p. 6). In the sense of "catering for the material and other general well-being of the one receiving care" (Lynch & McLaughlin 1995, p. 256), medical travel facilitators in Delhi are actively engaged in caring *for* international patients. Of course this is not always the case, but drawing on the data collected in the scope of this study, the manner in which most medical travel facilitators care for their patients seems to meet the virtues of attentiveness, responsiveness and respect emphasized by Engster (2005), complemented by commitment and emotional engagement discussed by Lynch and Walsh (2009). Exactly because of the "emotional work and moral commitment" (Lynch & Walsh 2009, p. 42), that the participants of this study convey suggests that medical travel facilitators not only care *for* international patients but also care *about* them.

CARING *ABOUT* INTERNATIONAL PATIENTS

Lynch and McLaughlin (1995, pp. 256–257) describe caring *about* somebody as "having affection and concern for the other and working on the relationship between the self and the other to ensure the development of the bond." In contrast to caring *for*, which is more practically orientated, caring *about* draws on emotional aspects involved in care. One of the main pillars of caring *about* according to Lynch and McLaughlin (1995, pp. 256–257) is relationship building and bonding, which indeed turned out to be a crucial aspect of medical travel facilitation in Delhi. So, how does the relationship between patients and facilitators develop? Just as Tariq and his patients do in that hospital in central Delhi, many times patients, their attendants and medical travel facilitators spend the whole day together and thus often share their daily routines. They begin the day together in the morning, go to the hospital to do the investigations, have lunch together, continue with their program, have a coffee in the afternoon and leave the hospital at the end of the day, sometimes they even have dinner together. Facilitators and patients also undertake activities outside the hospitals such as doing some shopping or sightseeing, taking daytrips out of Delhi or celebrating seasonal festivities. Starting from a customer-client relationship, the contact between facilitators, patients, and attendants is thus often extended to several dimensions of their private and social life.

Not uncommonly, the relationship that unfolds between facilitators and patients is marked more by a sense of friendship and familiarity rather than by a commercial undertone. The interviewees usually refer to the people to whom they provide their services as "their patients" but according to the situation they also use affectionate names like "my friend," "my brother" or "my uncle," even if there is no kinship between them. The use of these words reflects the facilitators' perception of the relation as being "more of a personal relationship than a professional one," as one of the interviewees points out. The frequent use of possessive pronouns to refer to "their" patients further indicates a sense of belongingness and affectionate respect. One of the interviewee explains: "you are not just a facilitator, translator or interpreter for that person who is coming from far away. You are like his family member" and another one rewrites his position as being basically "the first alien family member" in the patient's kindred. Also, the following quote reflects that facilitators consider their relationship with patients as much more than a mere business relationship and more than friendship even: "Not on business base. You know, I am not just translator, you know? I'm feeling they are just like my family. For that I am requesting, helping them. I'm doing my best. Okay? For that it is not business, not just friend. I'm feeling that they are my family, real family." The facilitator expresses commitment and devotion in doing her best to help the patients with whom she feels closely related and about whom she is emotionally concerned. This quote shows that the interviewees not only report that their patients articulate them as being like family members but that facilitators too use the same allegory by taking their patients as their family members, which indicates mutual attachment which is a common feature of caring relations. A sense of mutuality, belongingness, and emotional attachment is well reflected in the statements of an interviewee who uses the metaphor of a marriage: "So it is a marriage, every patient that we serve, we are married to that patient throughout his life." This metaphor alludes to a strong bond between two parties who are both committed to their relationship over a long period of time. Consistent with the metaphor of family ties that last for a lifetime, the relationship between the facilitator and the patient are often maintained after the patients return to their home country. They keep in touch over distance via phone or email and not uncommonly there is the opportunity for a reunion at a later time. One facilitator who is mainly serving Nigerian patients proudly explains that whenever he goes to Nigeria to meet with business partners, he feels like he is coming home because of the warm welcome he receives from his "friends" living there. These "friends" to whom he refers are former patients who are seizing an opportunity to express their gratitude by inviting him to stay at their houses or at least share a meal with their families.

Having affection and being concerned is another important aspect of caring about somebody (Lynch & McLaughlin 1995, pp. 256–257). Having affection goes along with building friendships and family-like connections. Narratives that evoke compassion and make the facilitators feeling emotionally attached to the patients they assist may also prompt affection and concern. When spending time together, common issues to talk about are the patients' situations back home, their struggle to access healthcare, the problems they face in raising money to afford the treatment abroad and the desperation that has resulted from these difficulties. Such emotive issues make the interviewees sympathize with their patients. Repeatedly they use rhetorical questions when reporting situations in which they are confronted with the patients' despair and predicament as in the following quote: "She is an old woman. So, if she is crying in front of you, what will you do at that time?" Such questions are taken as an indication that the facilitators themselves are sometimes overwhelmed by the situation and the complex emotional dimension involved in their work. The woman who openly displays her desperation and starts crying arouses compassion and draws in the interviewee helping her. Helping people in dire need seems to be considered as a moral obligation by some of the participants. Emotional attachment is then presented as a natural consequence of engaging with someone: "After all it's a human being, so you try to understand and learn something from them [international patients] and you will get some more attached and emotional." Being concerned is a feeling of being interested in and caring about a person which goes along with feelings of solicitude and responsibility that make that the concerned person becomes involved (Websters' Encyclopedic Dictionary 1994, p. 304). Medical travel facilitators may express their concern in a whole range of gestures, questions, actions, and advice that may seem insignificant at first glance but contribute to the overall well-being of the patients. Reminding them to wear a warm jumper like a concerned mother, giving them a hug like a brother, or making jokes to cheer them up as an old friend would do can evoke a sense of being well-guarded.

The interviewees seem to be especially concerned about the emotional state of international patients. Therefore, they support them emotionally in several ways and try to counteract their emotions and feelings of worry and anxiety, of insecurity and mistrust. In order to ensure the patients mental well-being, medical travel facilitators often engage in emotion work. According to Hochschild (1979, p. 561) emotion work is "the act of trying to change in degree or quality an emotion or feeling." Such a management of emotions or the influence upon emotional states, respectively, can happen "by the self upon the self, by the self upon others, and by others upon oneself" (Hochschild 1979, p. 562). When such emotion work is carried out in a commercial context, Hochschild (1983, p. 7) refers to it as emotional labor, which is the "management of feeling to create a publicly observable facial and bodily display." Such emotional labor is carried out by medical travel facilitators striving to give their patients a feeling of being in good hands and well cared for by an amiable facilitator, evoking positive emotions, radiating optimism, and counteracting the patients' anxieties and worries. Hence, facilitators are engaged in reassuring their patients that they have made the right decision coming to this particular hospital and that everything will be fine: "Hundred time we are telling you will be good and don't worry. This is the good hospital, you choose the best one, the doctor is very good. He will take care about you. So, we have to encourage them." Encouraging phrases offer comfort and reassurance to the patients who may have difficulties coping with the emotional stress they are exposed.

In order to express, show and induce certain emotions, facilitators need to manage their own emotions. The management of emotions, also referred to as deep acting (Hochschild 1979, p. 562), can be stressful and demanding. The manager of a medical travel company explains that his employees are being trained to make patients feel more at ease by deliberately steering conversations and choosing unencumbered topics and encouraging them. This is in line with Hochschild's (1983, p. 147) statement that employers can "exercise a degree of control over the emotional activities of employees." Although employers can ask their employees to do emotional labor, Hochschild (1983, pp. 148–153) argues that the extent to which emotional labor is performed and its quality also depends on the character and motivation of the individual, the expectations of the care-receiver, and the situation given. The extent to which emotional labor is carried out by facilitators indeed seems to vary according to the care needs expressed by the patients or their desire for autonomy alternatively, and also according to the facilitators' attitudes, the given situation and their emotional connection with the patient, which can be intricate. Many interviewees express that building and navigating the relationship with patients and attendants is difficult and a challenging aspect of their work. They have experienced situations in which patients are moody and turn their frustration toward them. Not seldom they would receive calls in the middle of the night because patients and attendants have sudden queries, they are asked the same questions again and again or they are confronted with persistent mistrust toward their persona despite their efforts. Nevertheless, the interviewees explain, they try to be understanding and respond kindly to the requests irrespective of how they themselves feel about it. In teams consisting of several members, the case managers can also help each other out if there are patients and facilitators that do or do not feel comfortable around one another. Despite having conflicting emotions personally, making the patient feel well cared for and investing in the relationship with them was still articulated as being pivotal.

Another concept that is associated with caring *about* and emotional labor and that is equally difficult to assess is that of "love labour." Lynch and Walsh (2009, p. 44) differentiate love labor from general forms of care work by conceptualizing it as "not only a set of tasks, but a set of perspectives and orientations integrated with tasks" that "is undertaken through affection, commitment, attentiveness and the material investment of time, energy and resources" (Lynch & Walsh 2009, p. 42). The facilitators' practices to care about their patients just outlined resonate with several aspects of this understanding. Considering patients as their friends or even as family members expresses a particular orientation toward the people facilitators care about and this orientation shapes the caring tasks performed by facilitators and the manner in which caring is carried out. The virtues of attentiveness, responsiveness, and commitment are upheld by the interviewees and enacted in a tailored service, quasi-permanent readiness to respond to the patients' requests, in the acts of advocating on the patients' behalf, and committing to a care relationship. Being personally involved and permanently on call demands time, energy, and other resources. Being emotionally attached, several facilitators report to invest money from their own pocket to enable the patients to access the needed treatments. As several statements of the interviewees showed, the bond that is established between facilitators and patients through caring relationships can evoke a sense of belongingness and mutual feelings of familiarity to the patients and facilitators alike. Though many facilitators show attachment, devotion, and commitment to care about their patients in an affectionate and loving manner, the approachability and evaluation of the qualities, intensity, and profoundness of the feelings involved and thus whether they actually do love labor is clearly limited. What is important, nevertheless, is to contextualize the care work carried out by medical travel facilitators within the industry that provides the setting thereof. The next section thus takes a critical look of the ambivalent rationales that underpin the facilitator's engagement in care.

UNRAVELING AMBIVALENT RATIONALES: BUSINESS STRATEGY AND SYMPATHY

So far, this chapter has elaborated different ways of conceptualizing medical travel facilitation in Delhi as caring *for* and caring *about* international patients. Now it is time to situate these practices in the business context in which most of that facilitation work is carried out as it brings ambivalent rationales to the fore that may motivate facilitators into doing such care work. Medical travel facilitators earn a salary with their work, though the patients do usually not pay them directly. All the interviewees were tied-up with one or several private hospitals that issue commission fees for referring and admitting international patients. That this payment is a transaction between corporate healthcare providers and medical travel facilitators may obscure the commercial setting to some patients who are not fully aware of this business model. However, the question arises that the facilitators' commitment toward caring well for their patients may be motivated by business interests rather than sympathy with the individuals they are supporting onsite? It may be argued that facilitators purposefully craft the relationships with their patients in a particularly caring manner that fosters their business.

In order to elaborate this argument, word-of-mouth as an important mechanism shaping the medical travel industry needs to be introduced first.

Since word-of-mouth recommendation is a powerful marketing element in transnational healthcare, medical travel facilitators who want to sustain in their business are concerned with getting positive testimonials for their work. Whereas some studies consider the internet as a key driver for medical travel and one of the most important channels for medical travel companies to distribute information and promote their services (Lunt et al. 2010; Hanefeld et al. 2015; Snyder et al. 2012), the participants of this study all found that to them positive patient testimonials passed on by word-of-mouth constitute the most essential promotion channel. Word-of-mouth, conceptualized as an informal and personal form of communication, is an effective way of transmitting messages and in their study on medical travel to Malaysia, Yeoh et al. (2013, p. 196) found word-of-mouth a potent marketing tool since "most of the tourists were influenced by friends, family, relatives and doctor's referral." According to the facilitators interviewed in Delhi, detailed and authentic insights into medical travel provided by former patients best meet with the wish for trustworthy testimonials expressed by medical travelers. Some even argue that especially for the clientele they receive in Delhi, personal testimonials are highly rated. This results from the personal observations of some of the interviewees that patients from different regions employ different strategies to find a reliable healthcare provider: Whereas patients from Europe, North America or Australia are said to rely on numbers, figures, diplomas, and certificates, patients traveling from countries in the Global South are said to rather trust personal testimonials and recommendations. Given the power ascribed to word-of-mouth in this business, positive testimonials can boost medical travel and effectively promote medical travel companies and individual facilitator; negative testimonials, however, can harm the image of the industry and may end the career of a facilitator. The interviewees thus consider the establishment of reference-chains as an integral part of their work. Among other patient mobilization strategies explored in more detail in another contribution (see Hartmann 2019), it is worth to have a close look at the "patient testimonial mobilisation" strategy as it is closely entwined with the emotional and nurturing effects of the facilitators engagement in care work: developing a bond with international patients during their stay at the medical travel destination site and providing a fabulous experience may be part of the facilitators strategy "to win the hearts of the patients," as one of the interviewees says, and turning them into their ambassadors.

Since medical travel facilitators in Delhi rely on positive testimonials and personal recommendations, they seem to try hard to establish long-term relationships with their clients, as they are considered to be conducive for future business. This objective becomes apparent in the following quote: "This business is a word-of-mouth business. If you have a good experience with me today, you go and tell the people about me. [. . .]. And that's how my business will increase." As having a good reputation and being recommended to friends and relatives is vital for their business, medical travel facilitators are concerned with rendering a satisfying or even delighting medical travel experience. The all-round facilitation service complemented by practices of caring *for* and caring *about* the patients seems to be an integral part of this experience that eventually nurtures the clients toward his or her facilitator. One of the interviewees expresses that the relationship with the patients has a direct relation to his business: "I will deal with them like our family. So that is the reason why one patient come, one family, so through one patient, ten patients will come in the future." Caring for the patient as for a family member thus serves to explain why patients feel in good hands and recommend their facilitator. Depending on the facilitators' attachment toward the patients, acting like/ being a caring and concerned companion who provides emotional support is conducive to building relationships. Care, it is argued here, may thus work not only as a practice but also as a strategy with which to win patients as ambassadors who will enhance the facilitators' future business. Although there is certain ambivalence around the association of medical travel facilitation with the hospitality industry—most of the participants distance themselves from the formerly widely used but critical notion of "medical tourism," for example—the facilitators' self-perception as service providers as one of the prevalent understandings of their work (Hartmann 2017, p. 39–40) shapes the care they provide and how they think about it strategically. The earlier introduced notion of providing a concierge service illustrates well how medical travel facilitation draws on concepts of the hospitality industry that, in practice, involve different forms of care work, while at the same time (re)producing certain understandings of and expectations toward their work.

Nevertheless, the care medical travel facilitators provide seems to be also shaped by rationales of acting humanely, helping people in need and advocating in the interest of international patients. Even though care work may be part of their business strategy, this does not preclude authentic sympathy, concern, personal devotion, and attachment. This adds to the debate about whether or not and with what consequences care can be commodified (Folbre & Nelson 2000; Folbre 2006; Madörin 2009; Lynch 2007; see for example Hochschild 2003). In the case of medical travel facilitation in Delhi, it may be argued that non-commodifiable elements of care are provided in a commercial setting. Features like the other-centered character, mutuality, commitment, and more intimate feelings that Lynch and Walsh (2009, p. 51) consider as being of a non-commodifiable nature, are still reflected in some of the caring practices performed by medical travel facilitators. Although initiated by commodified caring relations in the sense of providing a service for money, such personal relationships in the sense of solidary bonds of friendships can arise that involve engagement in what is conceptualized as caring *about*.

The ways in which facilitators articulate both business strategy and sympathy as driving rationales for caring *for*, respectively, caring *about* international patients can also be linked to debates revolving around conflicting rationales in care work. In the article "For Love or Money—or both?" Folbre and Nelson (2000, p. 123) bring together "the world of money and profit and the world of care and concern." As it has been shown in the interviewees' statements, business strategy and sympathy both feature as rationales for carrying out care work and for building close relationships. The dichotomy between social and economic rationales, respectively, between love and money to express it more pointedly, does thus not necessarily apply to the realities on the ground. Business relationships may result in friendships and personal attachments may be conducive for business.

In this sense, business strategy and sympathy are articulated not as exclusive rationales but as coexisting ones. Furthermore, Folbre and Nelson (2000, p. 133) argue that external motivations like money do not necessarily undermine intrinsic motivation or caring feelings. The authors state that it cannot be argued per se "that markets must severely degrade caring work by replacing motivations of altruism with self-interest" (Folbre & Nelson 2000, p. 124). Accordingly, care work carried out by facilitators in a commercial context does not necessarily compromise the quality of the care work carried out. That facilitators are making considerable efforts to make patients feel comfortable by caring for them seems to be beneficial to both parties: International patients are being well cared for and supported in their needs and wishes and at the same time medical travel facilitators can foster their business with these practices.

MEDICAL TRAVEL FACILITATION BETWEEN BUSINESS STRATEGY AND SYMPATHY

This chapter sheds light on the work of medical travel facilitators who are making an important contribution to bringing transnational healthcare into being by mobilizing patients to the transnational market and turning them eventually into ambassadors of the industry. A close look at the practices of facilitators who are based in one of the main medical travel destination sites in India showed that the facilitation model practiced in Delhi excels in the comprehensive and individualized support of international patients onsite, whereby facilitators engage in a broad range of tasks (e.g., counseling, decision-making, coordination, guidance, translation, negotiation, cultural brokering, advocating, comforting).

Drawing on these empirical findings, this chapter explored how many of these practices can be conceptualized as care work. Drawing upon care work as a conceptual framework, it has been shown that these facilitators engage in multiple dimensions of care work such as physical, mental, cognitive, and emotional care work, though to a variable extent. What is especially notable about the medical travel facilitation model performed in Delhi is that facilitators are not only caring for the overall well-being of international patients but also express to care about them in a particularly concerned, devoted, and affectionate manner.

Secondly, it has been argued that care work may not only be a practice but may also serve as a business strategy. Depending on positive testimonials and personal referrals, facilitators seem to make special efforts in order to render a satisfying or even delightful medical travel experience and craft long-term relationships. Being / acting like a devoted caring companion thus helps to nurture patients and win them as ambassadors who will hopefully spread positive word-of-mouth that may increase future business.

Thirdly, the ambivalence produced by non-commodifiable care being rendered in a commercial setting has been elaborated on. The ways in which the facilitators convey the rationales of authentically experienced sympathy and of business strategy regarding their caring efforts indicate that these rationales are not exclusive but often closely entwined. Out of the commercial relation between facilitators and patients, personal relationships can develop. Medical travel facilitators may thus care for international patients as economic actors, and at the same time, they may also care about them as social actors. As Lynch and McLaughlin say, "'caring about' itself can be developed within commodified 'caring for' relations" (1995, p. 257). Thus, the dichotomy between social and economic rationales that is often presented in theory does not necessarily apply to the realities on the ground.

NOTE

1. All names changed.

REFERENCES

Bell, D. et al. (2015): Transnational healthcare, cross-border perspectives. *Social Science & Medicine*, 124, pp. 284–289.

Blouin, C., Drager, N. & Smith, R. (2006): *International Trade in Health Services and the GATS. Current Issues and Debates.* Washington, DC: The World Bank.

Botterill, D., Pennings, G. & Mainil, T. (2013): *Medical Tourism and Transnational Health Care*, D. Botterill, G. Pennings, & T. Mainil, eds., New York: Palgrave Macmillan.

Casey, V. et al. (2013): "You're dealing with an emotionally charged individual...": an industry perspective on the challenges posed by medical tourists' informal caregiver-companions. *Globalization and Health*, 9(31), pp. 1–12.

Connell, J. (2013): Contemporary medical tourism: Conceptualisation, culture and commodification. *Tourism Management*, 34, pp. 1–13.

Connell, J. (2015): From medical tourism to transnational health care? An epilogue for the future. *Social Science & Medicine*, 124, pp. 398–401.

Connell, J. (2006): Medical tourism: Sea, sun, sand and ... surgery. *Tourism Management*, 27(6), pp. 1093–1100.

Connell, J. (2011): *Medical Tourism*. Wallingford: CABI Publishing.

Crooks, V.A. et al. (2011): Promoting medical tourism to India: Messages, images, and the marketing of international patient travel. *Social science & medicine*, 72(5), pp. 726–732.

Crooks, V.A. et al. (2010): What is known about the patient's experience of medical tourism? A scoping review. *BMC Health Services Research*, 10(1), pp. 1–12.

Dalstrom, M. (2013). Medical travel facilitators: connecting patients and providers in a globalized world. *Anthropology & Medicine*, 20(1), pp. 24–35.

Dawn, S. & Pal, S. (2011): Medical tourism in India: issues, opportunities and designing strategies for growth and development. *Zenith. International Journal of Multidisciplinary Research*, 1(3), pp. 185–202.

England, P. & Folbre, N. (1999): The cost of caring. *The Annals of the American Academy*, 43(9), pp. 39–51.

Engster, D. (2005): Rethinking Care Theory: The Practice of Caring and the Obligation to Care. *Hypatia*, 20(3), pp. 50–74.

FICCI. (2017): *Medical Value Travel in India: A Value Driven and Patient Centric initiative*, Bangalore: Federation of Indian Chambers of Commerce and Industry.

Folbre, N. (2006): Measuring Care: Gender, Empowerment, and the Care Economy. *Journal of Human Development*, 7(2), pp. 183–199.

Folbre, N. & Nelson, J. A. (2000): For Love or Money—Or Both? *The Journal of Economic Perspectives*, 14(4), pp. 123–140.

Gan, L. L. & Frederick, J. R. (2011): Medical tourism facilitators: Patterns of service differentiation. *Journal of Vacation Marketing*, 17(3), pp. 165–183.

Green, M. & Lawson, V. (2011): Recentring care: interrogating the commodification of care. *Social & Cultural Geography*, 12(6), pp. 639–654.

Sen Gupta, A. (2015): Medical tourism in India: winners and losers. *Indian Journal of Medical Ethics*, 5(1), pp. 4–5.

Hanefeld, J. et al. (2015): Why do medical tourists travel to where they do? The role of networks in determining medical travel. *Social Science and Medicine*, 124, pp. 356–363.

Hartmann, S. (2019): Mobilising patients towards transnational healthcare markets—insights into the mobilising work of medical travel facilitators in Delhi. *Mobilities*, 14(1), pp. 71–86.

Hartmann, S. (2017): *The Work of Medical Travel Facilitators: Caring For and Caring About International Patients in Delhi*. Heidelberg, Berlin: CrossAsia-eBooks.

Hazarika, I. (2010): Medical tourism: Its potential impact on the health workforce and health systems in India. *Health Policy and Planning*, 25(3), pp. 248–251.

Herrick, D. M. (2007): *Medical Tourism: Global Competition in Health Care*. NCPA Policy Report No. 304. National Center for Policy Analysis, Dallas.

Hochschild, A. R. (1979): Emotion Work, Feeling Rules, and Social Structure. *American Journal of Sociology*, 85(3), pp. 551–575.

Hochschild, A. R. (1983): *The Managed Heart. Commercialization of Human Feeling*, Berkley, Los Angeles, London: University of California Press.

Hochschild, A. R. (2003): *The Managed Heart. Commercialization of Human Feeling*, 20th Anniversary Edition, Berkley, Los Angeles, London: University of California Press.

Kaspar, H. (2015): Private hospitals catering to foreigners underestimate interpreters' role. *Hindustan Times, published online:* http://www.hindustantimes.com/analy sis/private-hospitals-catering-to-foreigners-underestimate-interpreters-role/article1 -1333370.aspx, (accessed: 14.5.2015).

Kaspar, H. & Reddy, S. (2017): Spaces of connectivity: The formation of medical travel destinations in Delhi National Capital Region (India). *Asia Pacific Viewpoint*, 58(2), pp. 228–241.

Kingsbury, P. et al. (2012): Narratives of emotion and anxiety in medical tourism: on State of the Heart and Larry's Kidney. *Social & Cultural Geography*, 13(4), pp. 361–378.

Lunt, N., Hardey, M. & Mannion, R. (2010): Nip, Tuck and Click: Medical Tourism and the Emergence of Web-Based Health Information. *The Open Medical Informatics Journal*, 4, pp. 1–11.

Lunt, N. & Mannion, R. (2014): Patient mobility in the global marketplace: a multidisciplinary perspective. *International journal of health policy and management*, 2(4), pp. 155–157.

Lynch, K. (2007): Love labour as a distinct and non-commodifiable form of care labour. *Sociological Review*, 55(3), pp. 550–570.

Lynch, K. & McLaughlin, E. (1995): Caring Labour and Love Labour. In P. Clancy, ed. *Irish Society: Sociological Perspectives*. Dublin: Institute of Public Administration, pp. 250–292.

Lynch, K. & Walsh, J. (2009): Love, Care and Solidarity: What Is and Is Not Commodifiable. In K. Lynch, J. Baker, & M. Lyons, eds. *Affective Equality. Love, Care and Injustice*. Basingstoke: Palgrave Macmillan, pp. 35–54.

Madörin, M. (2009): Beziehungs- oder Sorgearbeit? Versuch einer Orientierung. *Olympe. Feministische Arbeitshefte zur Politik*, 30(10), pp.66–69.

Madörin, M. (2013): Die Logik der Care-Arbeit - Annäherung einer Ökonomin. In R. Gurny & U. Tecklenburg, eds. *Arbeit ohne Knechtschaft. Ein Denknetz-Buch*. Zürich: Edition 8, pp. 128–145.

Mainil, T. et al. (2012): Transnational health care: from a global terminology towards transnational health region development. *Health Policy*, 108(1), pp. 37–44.

Mohamad, W.N., Omar, A. & Haron, M.S. (2012): The Moderating Effect of Medical Travel Facilitators in Medical Tourism. *Procedia—Social and Behavioral Sciences*, 65, pp. 358–363.

Ormond, M. (2014): Navigating international medical travel: A three-country study of medical travel facilitators sending patients to Malaysia. In *ISA Annual Conference, Yokohama*. Yokohama: unpublished lecture).

Ormond, M. (2013): Neoliberal Governance and International Medical Travel in Malaysia. In J. Connell, L. Kong, & J. Lea, eds. *Routledge Pacific Rim Geographies*. Routledge Taylor & Francis Group, pp. 1–19.

Ormond, M., Holliday, R. & Jones, M. (2014): Navigating international medical travel: A three-country study of medical travel facilitators sending patients to Malaysia. In *ISA Annual Conference (unpublished lecture)*.

Ormond, M., & Lunt, N. (2020): Transnational medical travel: patient mobility, shifting health system entitlements and attachments, *Journal of Ethnic and Migration Studies*, 46:20, 4179–4192.

Ormond, M. & Sulianti, D. (2017): More than medical tourism: lessons from Indonesia and Malaysia on South–South intra-regional medical travel. *Current Issues in Tourism*, 20(1), pp. 94–110.

Razavi, S. (2007): The Political and Social Economy of Care in a Development Context. Conceptual Issues, Research Questions and Policy Options. *Gender and Development Program Paper Number 3, United Nations Research Institute for Social Development*, pp. 20–21.

Reddy, S. & Qadeer, I. (2010): Medical Tourism in India: Progress or Predicament? *Economic & Political Weekly*, XLV(20), pp. 69–75.

Smith, K. (2012): The problematization of medical tourism: a critique of neoliberalism. *Developing World Bioethics*, 12(1), pp. 1–8.

Snyder, J. et al. (2012): Medical Tourism Facilitators: Ethical Concerns about Roles and Responsibilities. In J. Hodges, L. Turner, & A. Kimball, eds. *Risks and Challenges in Medical Tourism: Understanding the Global Market for Health Services*. Praeger, pp. 1–24.

Snyder, J. et al. (2011): The "patients physician one-step removed": The evolving roles of medical tourism facilitators. *Journal of medical ethics*, 37(9), pp. 530–534.

Sobo, E.J., Herlihy, E. & Bicker, M. (2011): Selling medical travel to US patient-consumers: the cultural appeal of website marketing messages. *Anthropology & Medicine*, 18(1), pp. 119–136.

Wagle, S. (2013): Web-based medical facilitators in medical tourism: the third party in decision-making. *Indian Journal of Medical Ethics*, X(1), pp. 28–33.

Websters' Encyclopedic Dictionary (1994): *Webster's Encyclopedic Unabridged Dictionary of the English Language*. New York, Avenel: Gramercy Books.

Whittaker, A. (2015): "Outsourced" patients and their companions: stories from forced medical travellers. *Global Public Health*, 10(4), pp. 485–500.

Whittaker, A., Manderson, L. & Cartwright, E. (2010): Patients without borders: understanding medical travel. *Medical Anthropology*, 29(4), pp. 336–343.

Whittaker, A. & Speier, A. (2010): "Cycling overseas": care, commodification, and stratification in cross-border reproductive travel. *Medical Anthropology*, 29(4), pp. 363–383.

Yeoh, E., Othman, K. & Ahmad, H. (2013): Understanding medical tourists: Word-of-mouth and viral marketing as potent marketing tools. *Tourism Management*, 34, pp. 196–201.

Chapter 6

Giving and Receiving Help across the Border

Transnational Health Practices of Migrants in Finland

Laura Kemppainen, Larisa Shpakovskaya, Inna Perheentupa, and Driss Habti

INTRODUCTION

Recent research has highlighted the importance of transnational social ties and social spaces for the health and health practices of migrant populations (Villa-Torres, 2017). New digital technologies and ease of travel have created new opportunities for transnational involvement of migrants (Vertovec, 2001; Baldassar, 2007; Levitt, 2014) including transnational health seeking practices (e.g., Kemppainen et al. 2018; Lokdam et al.; 2016; Şekercan et al. 2018). Levit (2014) describes contemporary migrants' transnational lives as "keeping feet in both worlds," in their countries of origin and destination societies (see also Glick Schiller et al. 1992). Transnationalism is often associated with crossing geographical borders, but mobility is not a requirement for being transnationally engaged. Transnational activities may involve sending and receiving "things," such as goods and artifacts and exchange social remittances in the form of ideas and behaviors (Levit 1998; Vertovec 1999).

Contemporary societies are increasingly influenced by digitalization. The "virtual" transnational social space is facilitated by the new information and communication technologies and allows for easier communication and presence in multiple worlds at once (Baldassar et al., 2016; Wilding et al., 2020). Virtual social spaces are increasingly included in migrants' health-seeking and caregiving strategies as well. Research has shown that the use of digital technologies is an important part of transnational health practices especially for migrants who cannot travel back and forth to their countries of origin. These people rely on their migrant networks to access allopathic and traditional medicine or use telemedicine to gain services from their countries of origin (Gonzalez-Vazquez et al., 2013; Gideon 2011; Menjivar 2002; Tiilikainen & Koehn 2011). On the other hand, some migrants are "stuck in motion" because of their (il)legal status, which forces them to rely on informal and mobile health practices, such as buying medicine abroad or from informal providers and sharing medicine (Castañeda 2018).

Research on transnational health practices has primarily focused on medical travel. The aspect of the "movement of things," such as medications, commodities or symbols and meanings of health remain under-explored (Villa-Torres 2017; Kaspar et al. 2019). Kaspar et al. (2019) call the "multiple movements of health-related things and beings" as therapeutic mobilities, which includes movement of patients, nurses, doctors, but also information, narratives, gifts, and pharmaceuticals.

Our chapter draws on these discussions on migrants' transnational health practices and the new forms and ways of accessing healthcare and giving care to those who were "left behind." In this chapter, we concentrate on the movement of non-human things, however, acknowledging that it is often part of a wider assemblage of transnational health practices. We discuss the flow of things and ideas between the countries of origin and destination as a part of migrants' care seeking and caregiving strategies. Our case study examines transnational activities across the Finnish-Russian border. The different political and historical trajectories, welfare state models, health patterns, and consumer cultures of these neighboring countries create a fruitful context for studying therapeutic mobilities. Finland is a developed Nordic welfare state and an EU member state, while Russia has remained politically and culturally more distant from the EU countries. Health problems and levels of welfare are unevenly distributed across these countries, which can be seen in life expectancies, for example (see Lyytikäinen & Kemppainen 2016).

First, we are interested in Russian-speaking migrants who receive health-related medications, goods, advice and ideas from their country of origin without moving themselves or as in addition to their mobile practices. Second, we investigate transnational caregiving from both the "lay" people's and health professionals' perspective. Our data comes from two different projects: (1) interviews on experiences and practices of health with Russian-speaking migrants in Finland and (2) interviews with Russian-speaking physicians practicing medicine in Finland. To our knowledge, this is the first inquiry into the "immobile" transnational health seeking and care practices between Russia and Finland. Furthermore, there is less evidence of the transnational engagement of those "left behind" in Russia from the perspective of care (however, see Tiyainen-Qadir 2016).

Our results show that Russian origin migrants living in Finland look for and receive medical advice and medication from Russia and are engaged in care giving at a distance. On the other hand, the interviewed Russian origin doctors who have their practice in Finland are engaged in transnational care work by sending Finnish medications and medical advice to their relatives, friends, and colleagues in Russia. Thus, the flow of medical knowledge and medications is two-way. We argue that familiarity, trust, and social ties are an important factor shaping this two-way movement of transnational care. Patients on both sides of the border rely on their social networks in accessing care.

RECENT RESEARCH ON MIGRANTS' TRANSNATIONAL HEALTH-SEEKING AND CAREGIVING PRACTICES

Research on migrants' transnational health-seeking practices (or medical travel) has increased in recent years (Villa-Torres, 2017). Transnational health practices of migrants are associated with the barriers and limitations of the healthcare sector of their destination societies, such as cost, distance, language difficulties, and discrimination, but also with the perceived better quality of care and the economic capacity to pay for private services in one's country of origin (for reviews see Kemppainen et al., 2018; Villa-Torres, 2017). Often migrants are not looking for just more affordable care but also familiarity and more "affective" care (Lee et al., 2010; Sun, 2014; Main 2014). Furthermore, health beliefs and cultural preferences can push migrants to look for health services abroad (Lokdam et al., 2016; Şekercan et al., 2018). Research shows that migrants often use "hybrid" health seeking strategies, which include a mix of goods, ideas, and people between origin and destination countries (Hilfinger Messias, 2002; Seto Nielsen et al. 2012).

Increased transnational migration has led to the growth of transnational caregiving, when migrants find ways to care for their close ones and relatives at a distance (Baldassar 2007). From the perspective of social relations, this type of care can be seen as emotional and physical labor, care work, to support the close ones who cannot manage by themselves (Hoshchild 2003; Daly 2002). Transnational care often comprises of financial support and organizing hands-on care, but also moral support is an important part of it (Krzyżowski, Mucha 2014; Baldassar, 2007). Care work is a constitutive part of family and kin relations, but simultaneously it has low symbolic status as gendered invisible activity, which is naturalized and interwoven in female roles of being a mother or daughter (Jolanki, 2015a). Often the ones caring for their close ones perceive health care as not only physical work but also as moral support and expression of affinity and emotional attachment (Jolanki, 2015b). In transnational families, the intensive use of digital technologies is shown to contribute to strengthening ties and the circulation of cultural, economic, social and emotional resources (e.g., Madianou and Miller, 2012; Wilding et al., 2020). Digital technologies have created new possibilities for the long-distance coordination of the provision of care of the relative left behind (Baldassar, 2014) and they allow for the digital circulation of emotions, which "constitutes the mutuality of being that underpins familyhood at a distance" (Wilding et al., 2020).

Emotions are central in care, and an important part of the experience of the "therapeutic" (Kaspar et al., 2019). As Kaspar et al. (2019) argue "[A]s a (desired) effect, the therapeutic is an aspiration, a hope, a potentiality. It is an orientation towards the future, a future that is imbued with hope and hence of an affective/emotional texture." The authors argue that this affective side of the therapeutic has a strong mobilizing effect. Furthermore, previous research has highlighted how transnational ties and networks of care also involve a lot of emotional work and feelings such as longing and guilt (Boccagni & Baldassar, 2015). In general, recent research has started to pay more attention to the aspect of emotions in migration and to how emotions evolve and are negotiated in different settings, life circumstances and across distance and over time (Boccagni & Baldassar, 2015; Skrbiš, 2008; Baldassar, 2008). Migration, as a concrete move from a place to another, gives an interesting lens to study the social, cultural, and even material aspects of emotions as part of negotiating sense of self and belonging. We contribute to these discussions by describing how emotional ties, trust, and familiarity are integral part of our interviewees search for therapeutic medical encounters.

DATA AND METHODS

The data consists of two interview data: one with Russian-speaking lay people and the other with Russian origin physicians, who work in Finland. The first dataset collected in 2017–2019 consists of twenty-five interviews on health conceptions and practices of working age Russian-speaking migrants in Southern Finland. It was supplemented with two interviews from an ongoing data collection from project dealing with questions of cultural understanding of health and health activism. Participants were recruited through snowballing method using key informants of different ages and gender to diversify the sample. In total, there are seven men and twenty women in the sample. The oldest respondents are born in the late 1950s and the youngest in early 1990s. They have lived in Finland from one to nearly thirty years.

The second dataset of interviews with accredited and practicing Russian migrant doctors was collected in 2014–2015 as a part of a project on career mobility of Russian migrant physicians in Finland. It includes twenty-six interviews with physicians in different parts of Finland. Participants were recruited based on a list of registered physicians and supplemented with snowballing method. The sample includes twenty-two women and four men, which characterizes higher presence of accredited Russian women physicians in Finland (Habti 2019). Duration of their residence at the time of data collection varied between eight and thirty-five years. In both data, the interviews were conducted in Russian or in Finnish depending on the language skills and wishes of the interviewees.

Russian speakers are the largest foreign language group in Finland comprising almost 21 percent (around 79,000 persons) of all foreign language speakers (Statistics Finland, 2019). The two countries are geographically close and the Russian origin migrants take actively part in transnational practices (Kemppainen et al. 2020). Russian origin persons are considered to be less visible and culturally more proximal to the Finnish population than many other migrant populations (Liebkind and Jasinskaja-Lahti, 2000). However, there is evidence of discrimination against Russian migrants (Liebkind et al., 2016) and in 2011 survey around 10 percent of Russian speakers reported experiences of discrimination or unfair treatment in the Finnish health services (Kemppainen et al. 2018).

Russian origin physicians are the largest group of foreign origin physicians in Finland (Habti 2019, 86). The number of foreign-born physicians is still small but has increased fast in recent years. Finland has suffered from shortages of physicians especially in rural and remote areas and has started to recruit foreign-born physicians to resolve the situation (Kuusio et al. 2014). In 2016, there were 644 Russian origin physicians practicing in Finland (Habti 2019, 86). Internationally, the motivation for Russian origin doctors to migrate is shown to be better career expectations and quality of life in the destination countries (Habti 2019; Iredale 2012; Bradby 2014).

RUSSIAN ORIGIN MIGRANTS' TRANSNATIONAL HEALTH AND CARE PRACTICES

Finland as a Nordic welfare state offers universal healthcare to its residents who have citizenship or residence permit. All our interview participants have a legal status as residents or citizens, and thus, they have the right to receive low-cost public medical health services in Finland. Our previous research has shown that in 2011 around 15 percent of Russian-speaking migrants in Finland had traveled to Russia for healthcare during the previous twelve months (Kemppainen et al. 2018). The use of transnational healthcare was associated with lower integration to the Finnish society and experiences of discrimination in the Finnish health services. Similarly, many of the Russian-speakers interviewed for this study are engaged with medical travel, meaning that they travel to their country of origin for health services. Some travel especially for health services but others do regular health check-ups when they travel to their country of origin during holidays or for other purposes. Most commonly, they use dental services and private health clinics. However, some do not have possibilities or do not want to travel but are still engaged in transnational health practices, which do not require traveling. These types of medical encounters are often conducted over the Internet or by phone or include sending and receiving of medications, health products, and health-related ideas and information across the border.

Following earlier conceptualization of transnational health practices (Levit 1998; Vertovec 1999; Kaspar et al. 2019), we discuss two types of health practices: (1) Exchange of health-related information, beliefs, and habits and (2) Movement of health-related "things" (pharmaceuticals, health products, and technologies). We discuss these topics from the point of view of two-way process of receiving and giving care across the border.

EXCHANGE OF HEALTH-RELATED INFORMATION, BELIEFS, AND HABITS

Continuation of Familiar Treatment Methods and Health Habits in Finland

Studies show that migrants often carry with them health beliefs and traditions from their native cultures, which guide their health practices in the new host country (Bochaton 2019). Our data includes some interviewees who suffered from long-term health conditions and continued to treat them with familiar methods instead of turning to Finnish medical professionals. First example is Ksenia, a 30-year-old female, who had lived in Finland two years. She suffered from back pain, which had started some years before her migration. She preferred to treat her back with methods she was already familiar with, prescribed by a physician in Russia. At the time of the interview, she had never consulted a Finnish doctor, as she felt at unease with the Finnish healthcare system.

Ksenia: I practice yoga, and if the pain gets worse, I either give myself an injection, or ask an acquaintance to do it, or travel to St Petersburg, where they give it to me.

Interviewer: What kind of injections? Are they painkillers?
Ksenia: No, they are [drug name] vitamins, of course there are a little bit of painkillers too, [drug names]—homeopathic remedies, they help. I help my own organism, [drug names], they treat the intervertebral roots.
Interviewer: And a Russian doctor (prescribed them)?
Ksenia: In Russia, yes.
Interviewer: Did you consult anyone with this problem here?
Ksenia: It is expensive. I cannot do that at this point, because I do not work. I do not have an insurance. But if I had an insurance.

Ksenia explained that she did not visit the local physician, as she could not afford a Finnish insurance. Finnish public healthcare is based on universalist principles and all citizens and foreign citizens with a permanent residence permit are covered by the National Health Insurance, which also reimburses a small part of costs from using private health services (Vuorenkoski et al., 2008). Thus, the excerpt shows that Ksenia is not yet familiar with the Finnish healthcare system. Her hesitation might also stem from the negative experiences of other migrants who were denied preferred medical service or misunderstood the rules of its provision. The stories about somebody who respondents know or about "friends of my friends" who were not treated properly in Finland are circulating among Russian-speakers and are found in many interviews. However, if she was to visit a Finnish physician she would not be able to get prescription for homeopathic medicine, which is not considered as an official treatment method in Finland. In Russia, physicians more often practice complementary and alternative medicine, especially in the private sector, and can prescribe homeopathic drugs too (Sadykov, 2012; Brown 2008). Homeopaths in Russia are required to hold a diploma in advanced medicine and have a certificate demonstrating the required level of training in homeopathy (Sadykov, 2016).

A married couple, Sergei and Alina, who were recent migrants to Finland, told about a similar situation but this time with their son's treatment. The family had migrated to Finland in 2016. More than ten years ago, when they still lived in Russia, their son had been diagnosed with the gallstone disease and was prescribed a special diet. As the diet was effective, the parents had continued with the same diet after their relocation to Finland. They had familiarized themselves with the dietary restrictions and followed them strictly:

Sergei: Our older child has a gallstone disease. He has the stones in the gallbladder. He has the diet number five.
Alina: It is a very strict diet, this number five. The first time, when his condition got worse, he felt straight away cold, hungry, and weary. We learned to

prepare this diet very fast. We discarded a group of all sorts of bad (foods), corn, legumes. That is to say, that we have known this diet for many years.

Sergey and Alina refer to certain diet numbering, which was developed by the Soviet medical research institutions. Different diets included different sets of food and meal types recommended for particular type of diseases (Pevzner, 1985). Some physicians continue to prescribe these diets as a treatment or as an addition to official treatment in contemporary Russia. In Finland, the gallstone disease is seen as rare with children and usually if a patient is diagnosed with painful gallstones, they will be removed with endoscopy (Mustajoki 2019). Thus, if the family was to visit a doctor in Finland, a very different approach might be taken to their son's condition and treatment.

These examples tell about familiarity and preference of certain treatment methods, which migrants continue to use in their new destination country. Culturally meaningful care can contribute to one's sense of identity and community (Kaspar et al. 2019). However, the excerpts also show some problems, which migrants face in the new medical setting. Ksenia had misunderstood her rights for treatment in Finland and Sergei and Alina possibly had not looked for a second opinion for their son's health problem, which could be relatively easily cured.

Our findings resonate with what Castañeda (2018) has termed being "stuck in motion" when referring to migrants who feel trapped and unable to access health care because of their legal status. Often these migrants rely on buying medicine abroad, sharing medicine and prescriptions, and on informal providers. Whereas Castañeda's informants were "forced to seek healthcare that is improvisational and may pose additional risks" due to their citizen status (ibid. 30), in our data this "stuckness" on old habits and informal health care practices was connected to our interviewees' lack of knowledge or distrust in the Finnish healthcare system. Thus, such practices might increase the risk of their marginalization from the medical system in the destination society in the long-run. As these examples illustrate, these practices, which do not include travel, still include risks similar to the ones documented in studies on medical travel. Double medication or treatment, postponement of treatment and lack of follow-up and rehabilitation may have negative effects on patients' health and they may also create unnecessary costs for the healthcare systems (Lokdam et al. 2016).

Digitalized Information Exchange

Another prevalent theme in the interviews was online and teleconsultations with health practitioners in Russia. Some Russian clinics offer Internet consultation, which, for example, Elena, who was soon sixty years old, used mainly because she was dissatisfied with the Finnish physicians' diagnosis and treatment methods. She was very critical of the Finnish healthcare system and suffered from various health problems. During her thirty years in Finland, Elena had learned to navigate the Finnish and Russian health systems to find affordable, and more importantly, personally satisfying care and results. Often her frustration was with the Finnish physicians who did not give her exact diagnosis to her often complex and ambiguous health problems. In these cases, she either traveled to Russia or consulted online doctors to get a second opinion. Sometimes she took laboratory tests in Russia and heard about the results, diagnosis, and treatment advice via Skype or email.

For many interviewees, getting medical support in their native language was an important reason for transnational health practices. This was the case with Alina, who was in her forties, and whose older son's case was described above. Alina used telemedicine to get advice on her anxiety in her own language. Alina had survived a serious heart attack, which took long to recover. At the time of the interview, Alina suffered from a constant fear of a new heart attack, which she believed would kill her. Alina needed psychotherapeutic treatment to cope with her fear, but as she did not speak Finnish, she wanted to get the treatment in Russian. At first, she was provided with a Finnish-speaking psychotherapist accompanied by a translator, but according to her, the quality of translation was not good enough. She also felt that the Finnish-speaking therapists and nurses did not understand her. Alina's family could not afford a private psychotherapist. Instead, Alina consulted a Russian cardiologist, who she described as her "own doctor." The consultation took place both by phone and face-to-face when Alina visited St. Petersburg. Alina talks about the importance of having the treatment in her own language:

Alina: And when I see her in Russia, she makes corrections to my medical care, talks to me in a different way, explains the situation. She discusses with me. And here (in Finland), doctors do not do that with you. The chief director (of the International Cardio Centre) and, at the same time, my doctor. [—] She is a kick-ass woman, practicing surgeon. She says to me: you are young, you will recover. She gives me advice in life. [. . .] Here the psychiatrist does not talk to you, even if you feel absolutely horrible because of a constant fear of dying.

Alina's case illustrates that consultation and medical help in one's native language is especially important when mental health issues are discussed, and strong emotions are involved. Familiar language and the familiar doctor-patient setting creates more therapeutic atmosphere for Alina. Many other interviewees shared the view that in Russia doctors listen to the patient and take more holistic approach to treating them than in Finland. Similarly to Alina, also Katia preferred her psychological help and support in Russian, despite the fact that she was otherwise happy with the Finnish system, and had found "her doctor," whom she trusted from the Finnish private sector. When asked who she turns to when she feels unstable, she answers promptly: "I call my psychologist in Moscow."

In addition to calling and visiting Russia for Russian-language treatment, some of the interviewees had established Russian-speaking care networks of medical professionals in Finland. This was possible for those who were able to pay for healthcare in the private sector, where the patient has more possibilities in choosing the treating physician than in the public sector. For example, Natalia, who was sixty years old, presented herself as socially competent and well integrated to the Finnish society. She used Finnish private clinics, where she could choose the physician. Even if Natalia spoke Finnish well, having lived in the country already for twenty years, her "own doctors" were still Russian-speaking. She also had a Russian-speaking pharmacist acquaintance, to whom she turned on medical advice.

Besides consultations from the health clinics, online peer support is a common type of digitalized health practice. Russian-speaking networks in Finland and abroad were used for getting advice on different diagnoses and treatment methods. For example, Natalia felt that her friend abroad had been important in helping to find out what was wrong with her mother. She first tried to find an answer to her mother's changed condition from the Finnish public sector physicians, but they "had big problems with diagnosis" and could not find what was wrong with the mother.

Natalia: A friend of mine calls from America, and says: She has the Parkinson's. She said that to me at least ten times. Finally, I went to a private clinic with her [mother]. He also said yes [it is the Parkinson's disease].

Natalia had many friends from her university student times in Russia, who had immigrated to different countries around the world, and with whom she discussed daily issues and exchanged opinions and advice on medical issues. Krause (2008) defines these types of formal and informal contacts, which are used for finding support and help in finding the right treatment, as "transnational therapy networks." These networks are activated locally and transnationally in the event of sickness by consulting close ones and acquaintances about the treatment, cure, and recovery (see also Bochaton 2019). These types of networks were typical among our interviewees too.

Besides social networks, some interviewees searched for information in Russian-language web pages. Maria, who was in her forties, and had moved to Finland almost 20 years ago, used the Internet to search for a diagnosis for her child. Maria was certain that her daughter had autism, but despite her long-time efforts, she did not get diagnosis for her in Finland. During the period of uncertainty, Maria sought for information regarding autism online, and found some of the webpages of Russian NGOs working with autism especially useful, as they were translating the very latest knowledge on autism from English to Russian. The information she found on these web pages convinced her that her daughter had autism.

Interviewer: What is the situation with this [autism] in Russia?
Maria: It is very hard to live there, even for a healthy person. There is a lot I do not like in Russia, but what I do like, even if the state does not help people and kids with special needs, is that during the last five to seven years the non-governmental organizations are growing. They offer help, develop things, and look for financial possibilities and so on. In the beginning, this was where I found information in Russian, because one thing that they are developing is the translations from American sources into Russian language.

Web pages of the Russian non-governmental organizations provided Maria with Russian-language information on autism that she could not find in Finland. Recently she also found her way to a Russian-language NGO in Finland, which has started Russian-language peer-support groups for various diseases. Their aim is to translate and provide Russian-speakers with information from Finnish NGOs and support networks for different health conditions and illnesses.

Others also relied on Internet advice even on more serious health conditions, as Irina with her cancer diagnosis. At the time of the interview, Irina had gone through a series of cancer treatments. She appreciated Finnish specialized healthcare very much, but she was concerned with what she called over-medication, people using unnecessary drugs. Irina followed a retired Russian physician on the Internet. This physician published video lectures and writings on alternative medicine, such as treating several conditions with hydrogen peroxide and soda (bicarb). Irina trusted him, because he was retired and thus "not obliged to prescribe all kinds of medicines as the corrupted doctors today." By this Irina was referring to how the doctors were paid by the pharmaceutical companies. At first, having received her diagnoses in Finland, Irina tried to refuse from chemo and radiation therapy, as she had read online that these treatments were fatal. Her Finnish physician then sent her to a psychiatrist. According to Irina, the Finnish physician had told her boyfriend that "she (Irina) is in some sort of psychosis because she has read so much about chemotherapy online." After consultation with the psychiatrists, Irina started cancer treatments, and was, by the time of the interview, cancer free. Thus, the Internet provided some interviewees with familiar types of care and peer-support in their own language but included similar risks to medical travel—possible postponement of treatment, misinformation and possible double or conflicting treatment (Lokdam 2016).

Care Flows from Finland to Russia

Transnational care relations and flow of ideas and information worked also the other way round—from Finland to Russia. Those respondents, who had left behind aging parents in Russia, would typically worry about their health condition back in Russia, and try to enhance their parents' health by sharing advice on healthy living. This took place via telephone or the Internet, as the respondents could not visit their parents in Russia on regular basis. For example, Ksenia tried to affect her father's drinking habits:

Ksenia: My dad drinks a lot. I tell him, dad, don't drink, you will have diabetes. He smokes, and I tell him not to, as he will have problems with his lungs, but he does not listen to me. My grandmother found out that she has diabetes a while ago, even if we all told her to eat less sweets and fried food, and to eat more greens, she does not listen.

Vera had quite similar challenges with her aging parents:

Vera: Recently they have had a lot of problems with health. My dad smokes a lot, which does not improve his health. He has problems with his heart. They both have heightened blood sugar, which they are now monitoring. [—]
Interviewer: Do you influence their way of life somehow?
Vera: I would like to, because they complain, and I try to help. For example, I send money. But often they do not listen to me, I try to participate, but they are passive themselves.

For Vera and Ksenia, these discussions with their parents on health issues and their attempts to persuade them to keep a healthy lifestyle present a form of care work at a distance, in the situation when they are not able to take part personally in their parents' daily life. Despite that women are usually considered to be more responsible for the care of the elder parents, in our data this type of transnational care work was mentioned by both men and women. While men stress more their financial support to parents (this will be discussed later), all respondents expressed their emotional attachment to parents through their worries about their health.

Another example of caring at a distance was Olga's case. She was in her late fifties and had lived in Finland from 1991. She cared for her old mother at a distance by monitoring her health condition daily by phone. Her mother's condition demanded constant home care, which Olga had organized during her visits to her hometown in the middle of Russia. Olga would also arrange doctor's visits to her mother via telephone:

Olga: She tells me what are the symptoms. It is not like this problem just arose but she has lived with it already for years, and I know what it [the problem] is. But if I do not know, someone has, let's say, some acquaintance, or a nurse, who has some education. I ask around for advice. That is how it goes.

Thus, even if Olga could not be present in her mother's life physically, they could share the everyday life very intensively, as she was actively present by phone and by organizing her mother's care. In this task, her transnational social networks played a big role.

Previous cases discuss the so-called "lay" migrants' health and care practices. Our second data set consist of Russian origin physicians who practice medicine in Finland. Several of the interviewed physicians discussed how they advised their friends, relatives, and colleagues in Russia. Most often, this was in the form of prescribing Finnish medicine and consultation about treatment, but also advising on how to find Finnish physicians. For example, Igor, a specialist in his fifties, discussed the increasing interest toward Finnish medical specialists by patients in Russia. Because of this, Igor had created a Russian-language Internet platform, which helped Russian patients in finding medical experts in Finland.

Furthermore, the Russian origin physicians living in Finland pointed out how they not only advised acquaintances but also their medical colleagues in Russia. Yulia, a specialist in her fifties, told that she communicated with former colleagues in Russia often and participated in gatherings of her medical school alumni. Also Marina mentioned that she frequently exchanged ideas concerning medical treatment with their colleagues in Russia:

Marina: Another colleague in Russia had a patient with peroneal paresis. He didn't get much help for that. I sent him pictures and all from here, how the leg must be bandaged so that it doesn't hang. It's everything, catching up with them but also professional exchange. Quite many ask how to get treatment in Finland. I send them information about doctors and phone numbers and tell what to do. Not often, but once a month I receive some questions.

Thus, migration does not only change the lives of the ones who migrate but also the people left behind are touched by their relatives and friends' migration and transnational lives. The flows of ideas and knowledge between the receiving and sending countries can promote changes in both places

(Vertovec 1999). This includes also ideas and values related to health and healthy living and medical knowledge, which are exchanged between the ones who have migrated and those who stayed.

Movement of Health-related "Things"

Movement of Medications and Health Products from Russia to Finland

Often the exchange of information was combined with the movement of things—mainly pharmaceuticals and health-related products. Anna, a woman in her thirties suffered from depression. She had lived in Finland more than ten years, was familiar with the public and private health system, and had studied nursing in Finnish. Originally, when she started to feel depressed she sought treatment in Russia, where she was committed to hospital, diagnosed with depression and prescribed antidepressants. She explained that she went to Russia because she felt she needed the treatment in her own language. However, after a while she wanted to renew her prescription in Finland and went to see a local physician. The physician told her that would need to start the diagnosis process from the beginning to be able to get a Finnish prescription. The physician explained that he did not want to take any responsibility for the medication prescribed by someone else. Thus, Anna continued to use and buy medication from Russia. She felt frustrated, as she already had a diagnosis and medication that she felt helped her but was difficult to acquire.

In addition to medicine prescribed in Russia, some of the interviewed Russian-speakers used natural products, which they knew from their countries of origin and which they regularly received from abroad. They asked their relatives and friends to bring natural products, such as herbal teas or Asian traditional medicines, from Russia or they bought them themselves when visiting Russia. For example, Irina explained how she used herbal tea and Tibetan medicine. She received these from her sister, who bought them from a local doctor in St Petersburg and brought to her to Finland. Another interviewee also received herbal teas from her sister, who brought them from Kazakhstan. The Internet had created new opportunities to find and order medication and health products online. In some cases, grown-up children who were accustomed Internet users helped their parents to buy traditional herbal medicine online from Russia. As Alex told about his parents who use quite a lot of different natural salves, which come from Asia and Far East:

Alex: I help them to order them online directly to here [Finland], since there is no representative office of these products here. Someone in Russia has recommended them [natural products] and they continue using it.

Herbal and natural products, vitamin therapies and homeopathy are widely used in Russia and many physicians prescribe these to their patients (Brown, 2008; Iarskaia-Smirnova & Romanov, 2008). Furthermore, the Internet and online Russian-speaking communities are used to sharing medicines and advice regarding its use. Tatiana tells about the cultural differences of using pharmaceuticals and health products as well as talking about one's health problems and sharing advice and medicine with friends and relatives.

Tatiana: In Russia, medical drugs are easily accessible without prescription, and everyone consumes insane amounts of drugs, and practices self-medication, because we have more possibilities. No one says, you have a cold, it will pass within a week. Medicine is being prescribed, bought, used, recommended, shared with friends. Russian-speakers do like this, just share the medicine. On the Internet, they are shared, discussed. But among Finns this is not typical. I had a Finnish acquaintance, and it was obvious, that she was tired, and then it became clear, that the person is truly ill, and on medication [but did not tell about it]. But my Russian acquaintances, when they wake up, they straight away share, if they feel pain today.

Thus, Internet created an important peer-support platform for discussing familiar medicine and its use. Sometimes these forums are also used for asking help in bringing different health-related products to Finland. However, as in other forms of transnational health practices, here too the risks are obvious, since recommending and sharing medicine without medical professionals' consultation can include several risks and be harmful for health.

Movement of Medications, Technologies, and Money from Finland to Russia

Even if some of the Russian-speaking migrants preferred to use Russian pharmaceuticals and herbal products, the quality of Russian drugs is often considered as low and counterfeit drugs widespread (e.g., Ozawa et al. 2018; Jeskanen 2020). Thus, Russian-speaking physicians working in Finland often prescribed Finnish medication to their networks living in Russia. Among others, Tania, a generalist in her thirties, and Yulia, a specialist in her fifties, wrote prescriptions for their relatives and acquaintances in Russia:

Tania: In Russia, I don't have contacts, except few rare contacts with people I know, professionals and acquaintances. Most often, it involves drugs prescription when people do not trust Russian drugs in order to avoid counterfeits.
Yulia: I consult relatives and friends from [two Russian cities]. Sometimes, I help them to buy medicine here.

Due to the low quality of some medical drugs sold in Russia, especially drugs needed for special health conditions, there is increasing interest toward medication available in Finland. The additional challenge is that special medication is expensive in Russia, despite no guarantees of it being good quality (see Ozawa et al. 2018; Jeskanen 2020). This is how Marina, a specialist in her late fifties, described the situation:

Marina: I know that in the hospital I worked in, in Russia, everything is going worse. I help friends there quite much. Everything is getting worse there. It's a bit hard to explain but during the Soviet Union, everything worked quite well, but when it broke up nothing was working. Before medication was free, but now you should pay when you get something. For example, my best friend's daughter in Russia has breast cancer, that's hard. They have to pay very much on their own . . . They ask me for advice. I write them prescriptions from Finland. They buy the medicines in full price, of course, but at least they know it is the right medicine.

Also Finnish private sector clinics have noticed the growing need for high-quality drugs in Russia. A Finnish private clinic has started an online service, through which Russian patients can buy prescription to Finnish pharmacies and courier service of drugs to Russia. According to the managing director of the company, most of the medicines are ordered for serious illnesses such as cancer. A prescription to a Finnish pharmacy costs 48 euros not including the price of the medicine, which is often much higher in Finland than in Russia (Jeskanen 2020).

In some cases, also medical technology had traveled across the Finnish-Russian border from colleague to another. According to Vladimir, a specialist in his fifties, there had been a shortage of technological healthcare equipment especially in the 1990s, and he had thus taken up the habit of passing on used medical technology from Finland to Karelia and instructing the local professionals how to use it. He explained this as humanitarian aid and as contributing with his expertise to the development of the healthcare sector in Russia.

Many interviewed "lay people" sent money to Russia for helping relatives to cope with their health problems. Many interviewees told that they frequently transferred money for their parents in order for the parents to use it for medical services in Russia. Thus, the parents were at times financially dependent on their children living abroad, as was the case with Maxim.

Interviewer: who can help your parents, if there are some necessities?
Maxim: Financially, only me [. . .] Physically, if something bad happens, I quit what I am doing here, and travel there instantly. It takes seven hours [to get there].

In some cases, financial support was offered as a compensation for the fact that the respondents could not travel to Russia often, and take care of their parents when they were in need of care or medical treatment. In these cases, care work at a distance included transfer of money for obtaining good quality care, such as health checks, treatment, surgeries, and other types of medical operations. This type of care work was especially important for the male respondents as they were less involved in other forms of organizing care. For some interviewees, feelings of guilt played a role and they tried to compensate their lack of presence by sending money or calling their parents regularly. They sometimes paid for the face-to-face care they could not give themselves because of the distance. This was the case especially, if the parent lived far from the Finnish-Russian border as in the case of Maxim, who instead of visiting regularly paid money to get her mother treatment in the best facilities.

TRANSFERRING "MEDICAL CULTURE" BETWEEN THE COUNTRIES OF ORIGIN AND DESTINATION

Recent research has shown that migrants assemble a mix of goods, ideas, and people between origin and destination countries, as part of their health-seeking strategy (Hilfinger Messias, 2002; Seto Nielsen et al. 2012; Kaspar et al. 2019; Krause 2008; Bochaton 2019). This "hybridity" is strongly present in our data too. Migrants mobilize "transnational therapeutic networks" (Krause 2008) in finding a good and trustworthy doctor and familiar treatment methods in the new medical setting. Often they rely on the networks and services of their own-language groups. These networks are also enacted to provide care for relatives and friends in one's country of origin.

Trust and emotional connectedness play an important role in navigating between the old and new practices of health. Strong trust in social networks can be seen as a form of historical *blat* networks familiar from the Soviet times (Ledeneva 2009). Ledeneva defines *blat* as "the use of personal networks for obtaining goods and services in short supply and for circumventing formal procedures." *Blat* can be understood as an exchange of favors and as the know-how of the (Soviet) system, and as a way to guarantee goods and services that citizens were entitled to but did not obtain. Furthermore, informal practices facilitated some personal freedom and choice in the rigid Soviet system. This social exchange of favors has been documented to continue in its more "monetized" form in the contemporary Russia too (Ledeneva 2006; 2009) and are enacted out in transnational context too.

In our interviews, the role of social networks appears especially important in finding one's "own" doctor, who is trustworthy. The interviewees preferred to have a "doctor of their own," either in the new country of residence or back in Russia. In some cases, the feeling of someone being "your doctor" was strengthened by the fact that the doctor spoke Russian. The will to have a doctor of one's own also echoes the importance of being understood and being able to use one's own language, which is a common motivation for transnational help-seeking. This discourse is familiar from research on Russian healthcare and medical culture. Lack of trust in the official healthcare system is shown to be typical for Russian patients (Aronson 2006; Zdravomyslova & Temkina 2009). In the public discussion, insufficient financing of the public health sector is seen as leading to the low interest and motivation of the physicians to provide qualitative care. On the other hand, doctors in private clinics are suspected of putting commercial interests before professionalism. Patients express their fear that doctors on private clinics prescribe more expensive treatment, more numerous and expensive medications than is really needed (Zdravomyslova & Temkina, 2008; Zdravomyslova & Temkina 2009; Chikirikova & Shishkin 2014). In this situation, finding a trustworthy doctor, with whom one can establish a personal relationship becomes crucial (Zdravomyslova & Temkina, 2009). Zdravomyslova and Temkina (2009) describe mobilizing social networks, consisting of relatives, colleagues, friends, and friends of friends, as an effective strategy in finding a doctor who is recognized as having a "good reputation," that is, who can be trusted. This institutionalized lack of trust and mobilization of social networks (*blat*) in finding a trustworthy doctor are prevalent features among the interviewed Russian-speakers in Finland too.

Another strategy by the more well-off Russian patients is to pay for the medical services in the private sector. In private clinics, patients can more freely choose their doctor, ask for specialist treatments, and participate in deciding about the treatment methods. In addition, informal payments to the treating physician are still a common practice in the healthcare sector in Russia. The informal payments help to build a trustful relation through a sense of control over the doctor's actions and the course of treatment (Brednikova, 2009; Temkina 2017). Choosing the private clinic is also a question of class. Ability to pay for the private service is considered as a sign of social identity and moral status (Rivkin-Fish, 2009; Shpakovskaya, 2015). This classed practice is documented in medical travel research too. Horton (2013), argues that medical travel is used as a way of "class transformation" when the income acquired in the destination country allows migrants to use private clinics in their countries of origin. In Europe, especially migrants from Eastern European countries tend to travel to their countries of origin to be able to use private clinics (Stan, 2015; Sime, 2014; Main, 2014). Being able to use private services and the "best doctors" is seen as a pride among the interviewed Russian-speakers in our study too. If our interviewees traveled for healthcare, they often preferred for private clinics. When travel was not possible, they used online health services offered by the Russian private clinics, which are relatively inexpensive with the Finnish income.

Zdravomyslova and Temkina (2009), describe another strategy, which is developed to navigate the untrusted healthcare system in Russia, which they call "self-enlightenment." Due to lack of trust, patients aim to become themselves experts in their illness and methods of treatment by obtaining specialized medical knowledge. Popular medical journals, professional medical literature, radio and television programs, and the Internet are all helpful resources for actualizing this strategy (Zdravomyslova & Temkina 2009). Furthermore, the Internet provides a community to exchange information about clinics and physicians, and to give advice on health issues (Bereguzova 2016). For example, women on parental web-forums compose lists and ratings of reliable fertility specialists, gynecologists, or pediatricians (Chernova & Shpakovskaya 2011). As we have shown, the Internet and social networks are actively used by Russian-speaking migrants in Finland too when they search for the health information and establish care relationships.

Migrants have transferred these ideas, ideals, and practices to their destination country. The interview data shows that many Russian-speakers did not completely trust the Finnish healthcare system either. Migrants are able to use their transnational cultural capital (Grineski 2011; Erel 2010) and, even more importantly, transnational social capital to navigate between different health systems and cultures: between the private and public sectors and across the border. Transnational networks were mobilized to find the best and trustworthy doctor and treatment method for oneself or to help a relative, friend, or colleague in Russia.

As the examples discussed in this chapter show, our interviewees were using digital tools in various ways in order to establish and maintain care relations at a distance. Digital technologies allowed them to endorse "the mutuality of being," which is important for maintaining the feelings of familyhood at a distance (Wilding et al. 2020) and a two-way flow of care, when necessary. Urry (2002) has argued that physical co-location cannot be fully replaced by digital co-presence, since physical proximity is necessary for some forms of social life. However, other mobility scholars have illustrated how there need not to be hierarchy between the physical or digital forms of co-presence—and that distant care is not necessarily less important than physical caregiving (Baldassar 2016; Madianou 2016; Wilding et al. 2020). Indeed, physical distance has even been shown to increase the efforts for care and expression of sentiment for those left behind via digital technology (Baldassar 2016). Our interviewees were in contact with their close ones, colleagues and friends in other countries on a regular basis, and communicating availability of support when necessary was part of their routine everyday lives. The digital tools supported their long-distance care relations. Thus, the cases discussed illuminate how the expanding amount of digital technologies available have not only brought new opportunities for migrants in "keeping their feet in both worlds" (Levitt 2014), but for creating new ways of caring for others and the self.

CONCLUSIONS

In this chapter we have explored the health practices at a distance by using interview data with Russian-speaking "lay" migrants and Russian origin physicians in Finland. We have shown that in addition to actual medical travel, also ideas, things, and even technologies move across the border. Often mobile and immobile practices were combined, but there were some interviewees who relied only on immobile practices. Furthermore, digital technologies are an important part of everyday care networks of the interviewed migrants. We argued that migrants create a hybrid of old and new ways of health seeking and habits and draw on both Finnish and Russian "medical cultures." Trust, familiarity, and feelings of obligation guide their navigation between the different systems and practices. Moreover, creating and maintaining "transnational therapy networks" (see Krause 2008), or *blat* networks, was an important part of our interviewees' health strategies.

As in the studies on medical travel, our study found that many of the described practices were associated with barriers of access, such as cost and access (especially in regards to access to private services), lack of trust and language difficulties. Trust plays an important role in our data and is often the main reason for looking for transnational medical advice and treatment. In addition to complex systems of trust, the importance of being understood and being able to use one's own language come forth as motivators for engaging with transnational health practices. Moreover, emotional reasons and search for a familiar and "therapeutic" experience were an important part of our interviewees' health practices. As Lee et al. (2010) argue, feelings of being "in-place," trust and familiarity are important in creating a sense of well-being (see also Kaspar 2019).

We have shown how trust and familiarity played a role in continuing with treatments and health advice prescribed in Russia and in engaging in long-distance advising from peers or medical professionals. On the other hand, the interviewed doctors felt a sense of obligation both professionally and personally to continue being engaged with the development of the healthcare sector of their country of origin as well as providing good quality advice and drugs to their friends and relatives who stayed behind. Similarly, "lay" migrants felt obliged to care for their aging parents and sometimes guilt of not being there for them. This guilt was suppressed by trying to keep in touch and to provide moral and, when possible, financial support for those who were left behind.

On the one hand, being able to navigate different systems of care and looking for the best suitable option for oneself can be considered as an act of resistance and to contribute to one's sense of agency and well-being. On the other hand, transnational health practices can be a sign of health and socio-economic inequalities as some of our interview excerpts suggest. Migrants can be "stuck in motion" (Castañeda 2018) because of several barriers of access to local health services and forced to rely on transnational health practices. Distrust toward the official healthcare sector and a sense of being misunderstood can lead to the underuse of services and act as barriers for service use (Akhavan & Karlsen 2013; Whetten et al. 2006). Furthermore, postponing treatment, the lack of after-care and follow-up, as well as wrong self-diagnosing or misunderstanding of one's treatment options can be detrimental to one's health. Thus, if lack of trust, higher price, language issues, or discrimination pushes people to seek healthcare from the Internet or abroad the question is of unequal or even discriminating system, instead of a therapeutic experience or choice (see also Kaspar et al. 2019). Transnational practices also raise a question of global health inequalities; who has the capacity to move or travel for better treatment or to healthier spaces? This is also prevalent in ordering high-quality drugs with high cost or getting to choose your "own" doctor in the private clinics.

REFERENCES

Aronson, P. 2006. "Utrata institutsionalnogo doveriia v Rossijskom zdravookhranii." *Zhurnal sotsiologii i sotsialnoj antropologii* 2, 120–130.

Akhavan, S., Karlsen, S. 2013. "Practitioner and client explanations for disparities in healthcare use between migrant and non-migrant groups in Sweden: A qualitative study." *Journal of Immigrant and Minority Health* 15(1), 188–197.

Baldassar, L. 2007. "Transnational families and the provision of moral and emotional support: The relationship between truth and distance." *Identities* 14(4), 385–409.

Baldassar, L., Nedelcu, M., Merla, L., Wilding, R., 2016. "ICT-based co-presence in transnational families and communities: Challenging the premise of face-to-face proximity in sustaining relationships." *Global Networks*, 16(2), 144–144.

Baldassar, L. 2016. "De-demonizing distance in mobile family lives: co-presence, care circulation and polymedia as vibrant matter." *Global Networks* 16(2), 145–163.

Bereguzova, E. 2016. "Rol' sotsial'nykh media v formirovanii praktik zaboty o zdorov'e sredi sel'skoj molodezhi." *Ekonomicheskaya sotsiologiya* 17(5), 103–129.

Boccagni, P., Baldassar, L. 2015. "Emotions on the move: Mapping the emergent field of emotion and migration." *Emotion, Space and Society* 16(2015), 73–80.

Bochaton, A. 2019. "Intertwined therapeutic mobilities: Knowledge, plants, healers on the move between Laos and the U.S." *Mobilities* 14(1), 54–70.

Bradby, H. 2014. "International Medical Migration: A Critical Conceptual Review of the Global Movements of Doctors and Nurses." *Health* 18(6), 580–596.

Brednikova, O. 2007. Pokupaya kompetentsiyu i vnimanie: Praktiki platezhej vo vremya beremennosti is rodov. In Zdravomyslova, E. & Temkina, A. (eds.), *Zdorovye i doverie: gendenyj podkhod k reproduktivnoj meditsine.* St. Petersburg: European University, 211–233.

Brown, S. 2008. "Use of complementary and alternative medicine by physicians in St. Petersburg, Russia." *The Journal of Alternative and Complementary Medicine* 14(3), 315–319.

Castañeda, H, 2018. Stuck in motion: Simultaneous mobility and immobility in migrant healthcare along the US/Mexico border. In *Healthcare in Motion: Immobilities in Health Service Delivery and Access.* New York: Berghahn, Books, 19–34.

Chernova, ZH, Shpakovskaya, L. 2011. "Politekonomiya sovremennogo roditel'stva. Setevoe soobschcestvo i sotsial'nyj kapital." *Ekonomicheskaya sotsiologiya* 12(3), 85–105.

Chirikova, A., Shishkin, S. 2014. "Vzaimodejstvie vrachej i patsientov v sovremennoj Rossii: Vektory izmenenii." *Mir Rossii* 2, 154–182.

Connell, J. 2015. "From medical tourism to transnational health care? An epilogue for the future." *Social Science & Medicine* 124, 398–401.

Daly, M. 2002. "Care as a good for social policy." *Journal of Social Policy* 31(2), 251–270.

Erel, U. 2010. "Migrating cultural capital: Bourdieu in migration studies." *Sociology* 44(4), 642–660.

Finnish Medical Association (FMA). 2016. Physicians in Finland: Statistics on Physicians and the Health Care System. Helsinki: National Institute for Health and Welfare. https://www.laakariliitto.fi/site/assets/files/1011/ll16_taskutil_06_en_160 524net.pdf.

Jolanki, O. 2015a. "To work or to care? Working women's decision-making." *Community, Work & Family* 18 (3), 268–283.

Jolanki O. 2015b. "Elderly Parents' need for help and adult children's move decisions." *Journal of Housing for the Elderly* 29, 77–91.

Gideon, J. 2011. "Exploring migrants' health seeking strategies: the case of Latin American migrants in London." *International Journal of Migration, Health and Social Care* 7(4), 197–208.

Glick Schiller, N., Basch, L., Blanc-Szanton, C. 1992. Transnationalism: A new analytic framework for understanding migration. In: *Towards a Transnational Perspective on Migration: Race, Class, Ethnicity, and Nationalism Reconsidered.* New York City: New York Academy of Sciences, 1–24.

González-Vázquez, T., Pelcastre-Villafuerte, B.E., Taboada, A. 2016. "Surviving the Distance: The Transnational Utilization of Traditional Medicine Among Oaxacan Migrants in the US." *Journal Immigrant Minority Health* 18, 1190–1198.

Grineski, S. 2011. "Why parents cross for children's health care: transnational cultural capital in the United States-Mexico border region." *Social Theory and Health* 9, 256–274.

Habti, D. 2019. "What's Driving Migrant Russian Physicians to Stay Permanently in Finland? A Life-Course Approach." *Journal of Finnish Studies* 22(1–2), 85–118.

Hilfinger Messias, D. 2002. "Transnational health resources, practices, and perspectives: Brazilian immigrant women's narratives." *Journal of Immigrant Health* 4(4), 183–200.

Hochschild, A. 2003. *The commercialization of intimate life. Notes from home and work.* University of California Press.

Horton, S. 2013. "Medical Returns as Class Transformation: Situating Migrants' Medical Returns within a Framework of Transnationalism." *Medical Anthropology* (32), 417–432.

Iarskaia-Smirnova E., Romanov P. 2008. Culture matters: integration of folk medicine in health care in Russia. In Ellen Kuhlmann and Mike Saks (eds.), *Rethinking professional governance: International directions in health care.* Bristol: The Policy Press, 141–154.

Iredale, R. 2012. Major Issues in the Global Mobility of Health Professionals. In Short, S., McDonald, F. (eds.), *Law, Ethics and Governance: Health Workforce.* London: Routledge, 15–40.

Krzyżowski Ł., J. Mucha. 2014. "Transnational caregiving in turbulent times: Polish migrants in Iceland and their elderly parents in Poland." *International Sociology* 29(1), 22–37.

Jeskanen, J. 2020. "Venäjällä paketti särkylääkettä maksaa 30 senttiä, mutta lääkkeiden laatu on romahtanut—helsinkiläinen lääkärikeskus alkoi kirjoittaa venäläisille reseptejä." *Helsingin Sanomat*, 10.2.2020. https://www.hs.fi/ulkomaa t/art-2000006401818.html

Kaspar, H., Walton-Roberts, M., Bochaton, A. 2019. "Therapeutic mobilities." *Mobilities* 14(1), 1–19.

Kemppainen, L., Kemppainen, T., Skogberg, N., Kuusio, H., Koponen, P. 2018. "Immigrants 'use of health care in their country of origin: the role of social integration, discrimination and the parallel use of health care systems." *Scandinavian Journal of Caring Sciences* 32(2), 698–706.

Kemppainen, T., Kemppainen, L., Kuusio H., Rask, S., Saukkonen, P. 2020. "Multifocal integration and marginalisation. A theoretical model and an empirical study on three immigrant groups." *Sociology*, online first, 54(4), 782–805.

Krause, K. 2008. "Transnational Therapy Networks among Ghanaians in London." *Journal of Ethnic and Migration Studies* 34(2), 235–251.

Kuusio, H., Lämsä, R., Aalto, A. M., Manderbacka, K., Keskimäki, I., Elovainio, M. 2014. "Inflows of foreign-born physicians and their access to employment and work experiences in health care in Finland: qualitative and quantitative study." *Human Resources for Health* 12(1), 41.

Ledeneva, A. V. 2006. *How Russia really works: The informal practices that shaped post-Soviet politics and business*. Ithaca, NY: Cornell University Press.

Ledeneva, A. 2009. "From Russia with *blat*: can informal networks help modernize Russia?" *Social Research: An International Quarterly* 76(1), 257–288.

Lee, J., Kearns., R., Friesen, W. 2010. "Seeking affective health care: Korean immigrants' use of homeland medical services." *Health & Place* 16, 108–115.

Levitt, P. 2014. Keeping feet in both worlds: Transnational practices and immigrant incorporation in the United States. In Joppke, C. Morawska, T. (eds.), *Toward assimilation and citizenship: Immigrants in liberal nation-states*. London: Palgrave Macmillan, 177–194.

Lokdam, N., Kristiansen, M., Handlos, L., Norredam, M. 2016. "Use of healthcare services in the region of origin among patients with an immigrant background in Denmark: a qualitative study of the motives." *BMC Health Services Research* 1, 1–10.

Lyytikäinen, L., Kemppainen, T. 2016. "Regional inequalities in self-rated health in Russia: What is the role of social and economic capital?" *Social Science & Medicine* 161, 92–99.

Madianou, M. 2016. "Ambient co-presence: transnational family practices in polymedia environments." *Global Networks* 16(2), 183–201.

Madianou, M., Miller, D. 2013. *Migration and new media: Transnational families and polymedia*. Routledge.

Main, I. 2014. "Medical travels of Polish female migrants in Europe." *Sociologicky Casopis* 50, 897–918.

Menjívar, C. 2002. "The ties that heal: Guatemalan immigrant women's networks and medical treatment." *International Migration Review* 36(2), 437–466.

Mustajoki, P. 2019. Sappikivitauti [Gallstone disease]. Lääkärilehti Duodecim. https ://www.terveyskirjasto.fi/terveyskirjasto/tk.koti?p_artikkeli=dlk00074. Accessed Feb 14, 2020.

Österle, A.J., Johnson, T., Delgado, Jose. 2013. "A unifying framework of the demand for transnational medical travel." *International Journal of Health Services* 43, 15–436.

Ozawa, S., Evans, D. R., Bessias, S., et al. 2018. "Prevalence and Estimated Economic Burden of Substandard and Falsified Medicines in Low- and Middle-Income Countries: A Systematic Review and Meta-analysis." *JAMA Network Open* 1(4): e181662.

Pevzner, M.I. 1985. "Osnovy lechebnogo pitania [Foundations of healing diets]." Moscow: Mediz.

Rivkin-Fish M. 2009. "Tracing landscapes of the past in class subjectivity: Practices of memory and distinction in marketing Russia." *American Ethnologist* 36(1), 79–95.

Sadykov, R. A. 2016. "Homeopathy within Russia Healthcare: The challenges of professionalisation." *Journal of Social Policy Studies* 14(4), 597–608.

Sadykov, R. A. 2011. "Drugie vrachi: puti professionlaizatsii predstavitelej al'ternativnoin meditsiny." *Sotsiologicheskij zhurnal* 2, 161–167.

Seto Nielsen, L.S., Angus, J.E., Lapum, J., Dale, C., Kramer-Kile, M., Abramson, B., Marzolini, S., Oh, P., Price, J. Clark, A. 2012. 'I can't just follow any particular textbook': Immigrants in cardiac rehabilitation. *Journal of Advanced Nursing* 68, 2719–2729.

Şekercan, A., Woudstra, A. J., Peters, R. J., Lamkaddem, M., Akgün, S., & Essink-Bot, M. L. 2018. "Dutch citizens of Turkish origin who utilize healthcare services in Turkey: a qualitative study on motives and contextual factors." *BMC health services research 18*(1), 289.

Shpakovskaya, L. (2015). "How to be a good mother: The case of middle class mothering in Russia." *Europe-Asian Studies* 67(10), 1571–1586.

Sime, D. 2014. 'I think that Polish doctors are better': newly arrived migrant children and their parents' experiences and views of health services in Scotland. *Health & Place* 30, 86–93.

Stan, S. 2015. "Transnational healthcare practices of Romanian migrants in Ireland: Inequalities of access and the privatisation of healthcare services in Europe." *Social Science & Medicine*, 124, 346–355.

Statistics Finland (2019). Official Statistics of Finland (OSF): Foreign-language speakers. Population structure [e-publication]. Helsinki: Statistics Finland [referred: 4.9.2019]. https://www.tilastokeskus.fi/tup/maahanmuutto/maahanmuuttajat-vaestossa/vieraskieliset_en.html

Sun, K. 2014. "Transnational healthcare seeking: How ageing Taiwanese return migrants view homeland public benefits." *Global Networks* 14(4), 533–550.

Temkina, A. 2017. 'Ekonomika doveriya' v platnom segmente rodovspomozheniya: gorodskaya obrazovannaya zhenshchina kak potreitel' i patsientka. *Ekonomicheskaya sotsiologiya* 18(3), 14–53.

Temkina A., Zdravomyslova E. 2008. "Patients in contemporary Russian reproductive health care institutions strategies of establishing trust." *Demokratizatsia* 16(3), 277–293.

Tiilikainen, M., Koehn, P. 2011. "Transforming the Boundaries of Health Care: Insights from Somali Migrants." *Medical Anthropology* 30(5), 518–544.

Tiaynen-Quadir, T. 2016. Transnational grandmothers making their multi-sited homes between Finland and Russia. In Walsh, K., Näre, L. (eds.), *Transnational migration and home in older age*. London: Routledge, 25–37.

Urry, J. 2002 "Mobility and proximity." *Sociology* 36(2), 255–274.

Vertovec, S. 1999. "Conceiving and researching transnationalism." *Ethnic and Racial Studies* 22(2), 447–462.

Vertovec, S. 2001. "Transnationalism and identity." *Journal of Ethnic and Migration Studies* 27(4), 573–582.

Vuorenkoski, L., Mladovsky, P., Mossialos, E. 2008. Finland: Health system review. *Health Systems in Transition* 10(4). European Observatory on Health Systems and Policies.

Whetten, K., Leserman, J., Whetten, R., Ostermann, J., Thielman, N., Swartz, M., & Stangl, D. 2006. "Exploring lack of trust in care providers and the government as a barrier to health service use." *American Journal of Public Health* 96(4), 716–721.

Wilding, R., Baldassar, L., Gamage, S., Worrell, S. Mohamud, S. 2020. "Digital media and the affective economies of transnational families." *International Journal of Cultural Studies* 23(5), 639–655.

Zdravomyslova, E. & Temkina, A. 2009. 'Vracham ja ne doveryayu, no...' Preodolenie nedoveriya k reproduktivnoj podkhod k reproduktivnoj meditsine. In Zdravomyslova, E. & Temkina, A. (eds.), *Zdorovye i doverie: gendenyj podkhod k reproduktivnoj meditsine.* St. Petersburg: European University, 179–210.

Chapter 7

The Dual Role of the Facilitator as Therapist and Reproductive Travel Broker in Cross-border Reproductive Travel from Developed Countries

Psychological and Ethical Perspectives and a Call for Separation of Services

Dr. Joyeeta G. Dastidar

One increasingly common scenario in reproductive travel is when a couple from a developed country goes overseas for in vitro fertilization (IVF). On the spectrum of assisted reproduction, and from the standpoint of the recipient (vs. donor) of reproductive services, sperm donation would be among the lowest risk interventions, and surrogacy among the highest risk interventions, with IVF or egg donation—both of which require ovarian stimulation and egg retrieval—somewhere in between the two. With IVF, a woman can use her own eggs, or, if with diminished ovarian reserve due to advanced age or other causes, may need to use an egg donor to supply the egg. The reasons for IVF-related travel are more varied and as diverse as the countries of origin of the women doing the traveling.

This chapter reviews the reasons couples seek IVF and more specifically IVF overseas as a basis to explain why couples from developed countries participating in cross-border reproductive care are especially in need of extra psychological support. Reasons for cross-border reproductive travel include a desire for anonymity presumably for sociocultural reasons, logistical issues such as restrictions on access to at home reproductive care based on age or insurance caps, financial reasons, as well as circumvention of laws in the home country, whether based on religion or a desire to protect more vulnerable populations. This variety of reasons presents quite the range of psychological and ethical concerns, with the two being intertwined at times.

These trips are often organized by facilitators, also known as reproductive travel brokers, many of whom concurrently fulfill the roles of providing emotional support to the couples pursuing cross-border reproductive care and of organizing that care by connecting the patient with an overseas institution +/- reproductive donor. The chapter looks at studies of couples traveling from Australia (to various countries) and the United States (to the Czech Republic) via the use of a facilitator. Beyond use of reproductive technologies with one's own gametes or sperm donation, reproductive travel brokers also facilitate use of egg donation, wherein they often are supposed to take on the additional role of protecting the egg donors. While each of these roles is essential, some are in conflict with each other, raising the question of how much a facilitator should really do, or whether the involved employees better serve their patients by a breakdown of their duties into distinct service providers. Furthermore, much could be gained by requiring some form of training and accreditation of the roles serviced by facilitators.

The chapter takes a look at the ways in which the role of facilitators or brokers can help offset the risk to participants in reproductive travel by paying attention to the need for care and psychological support by arranging for adjunctive services and adhering to quality control measures, including a review of guidelines emerging from various societies of reproductive medicine. The chapter ends with a suggestion for reconfiguring the roles fulfilled by the facilitator while maintaining the services offered to the patients.

REASONS WHY COUPLES SEEK CBRC

In their article *The ethical physician encounters international medical travel*, the authors G. Crozier and Francoise Baylis talk about patient decision spaces, which are the constraints (sociocultural, financial, legal, degree of medical necessity) within which patients make decisions about their healthcare. They note that physicians should look at the patient's case within this framework to determine when going abroad may be in the patient's best interest, versus when to actively discourage this (p. 298). The four broad categories of decision spaces encountered by physicians of more developed countries include (1) elective procedures expensive in the home country and available at a fraction of the cost abroad, (2) medically necessary procedures with long domestic waiting lists, (3) medical interventions not available in the home country because they have not been shown to be safe and effective, and (4) medical interventions unavailable in home country as there are legal prohibitions against them because they may harmfully exploit more vulnerable persons (p. 299). We should would add to this list fifth and sixth categories of decision space, (5) medical interventions which are safe and effective but not available in the home country due to lack of more advanced technologies, and (6) medical interventions available in the home country but underutilized due to social stigma whether in the society as a whole or for a particular sub-culture.

Applying Crozier and Baylis's notion of patient decision spaces to cross-border reproductive care demonstrates that at least four of these decision spaces come up: Couples travel abroad for cheaper IVF and/or egg donation. Couples from countries with national health services with long lists (e.g., Canada, the UK) often go abroad for faster access to the same services elsewhere. Countries such as Canada, Australia, and some European countries have banned egg donation and/or surrogacy due to concerns about the ethics of the practice as most often the reproductive donor is less well-off and more vulnerable. Other countries have similar bans based on religion (e.g., Islam, Catholicism). A fourth category is couples with infertility who live in the developing world that lacks IVF centers going abroad for reasons of access. A fifth category is couples going abroad for reasons of anonymity, whether due to social stigma of using IVF at home or wanting the gamete donor to remain anonymous.

FREQUENTLY EXPERIENCED PSYCHOLOGICAL EFFECTS OF INFERTILITY AND NEED FOR REPRODUCTIVE ASSISTANCE

Couples undergoing IVF are often committing to a series of tests and procedures repeated in cycles with the ultimate motivation of becoming a parent, often at the expense of finances, physical health, and time and driven by a vision of their future child. In their quest for parenthood, these prospective parents are driven by the quadruple motivators of hope, loyalty, love, and dedication (Vindrola-Padros, 2019, pp. 114–115, 122).

The optimal age for fertility is twenty to twenty-four. In much of the West including Europe and the United States, the average age for having kids is over thirty. While infertility is a medical condition, it is one that can have significant emotional and psychological consequences, with one study of infertile people indicating that 48 percent considered it the worst aspect of their lives. The stress from infertility can be akin to the stress of losing a loved one. The diagnosis of infertility is often met with denial, a loss of self-esteem, anxiety, depression, concerns about not being able to meet a partner's needs. Women and men have similar emotional reactions to infertility. Women may have more negative societal repercussions of infertility what with having children being seen as central to the role of women. Women can feel sad and uneasy about their infertility. Men on the other hand, associate their infertility with sexual function and this affects their self-esteem. Infertility can impact both one's emotional wellbeing and to a lesser extent, marital satisfaction (Malina and Cooley, pp. 555–556).

The start of infertility treatments often leads to a sense of loss of control over one's body. Given that IVF is one of the most effective forms of ARTs, one meta-analysis looked at the psychological impact of IVF as a way to guide social scientists given its significant impact on many individuals, couples, and families. Women are more studied in IVF, and from what we know, women also suffer greater negative emotional reactions to the process, including anxiety. Unsuccessful IVF attempts led to feelings of tension, sadness, anger, depression, helplessness, loss, guilt, and a loss of self-esteem. While possibly less intense, men also experienced similar feelings. Even with IVF success, couples tended to have more anxiety about pregnancies than fertile couples. The psychological effects on women were found to be long-term in a twenty-year follow up study, where women who underwent IVF had higher rates of depression, obsessive-compulsive disorder, and somatization, with women whose IVF experiences were unsuccessful even more likely to suffer from the mental health standpoint (Malina and Cooley, pp. 555–556). Perhaps this is due to the greater burden of testing and treatment on women, and the larger societal connotations of childlessness for women versus men.

Overall, two thirds of the studies looking at levels of distress and IVF treatment point to a negative effect, whereas the remainder show a trend, no effect, or did not gather enough data to address that question specifically. After realizing there were no validated scales looking at IVF and levels of distress, three researchers, Hillary Klonoff-Cohen, Loki Natarajan, and Elizabeth Klonoff developed a scale and validated a scale called the Concerns of Women Undergoing Assisted Reproductive Technology (CART; pp. 353–355). The best prospective data measuring the effect of stress and IVF came through the application of their scale through questionnaires administered at the first clinic visit as well as the time of treatment. They found that women concerned about the medical aspects of treatment had 20 percent fewer oocytes retrieved, and 19 percent fewer oocytes fertilized. Women concerned about missing work had 30 percent fewer oocytes fertilized and a 2.83 odds ratio against achieving a pregnancy. Women who were extremely concerned about the finances of IVF had an 11.62 odds ratio of not achieving a live birth (Klonoff-Cohen and Natarajan, pp. 983–986). This points to the need for pre-treatment education, support, and counseling to help lower stress levels before going into treatment. A later review found not only decreases in anxiety and depression but also increases in the rate of conception through support and counseling (Cousineau and Domar, pp. 298–300).

It is important to note that in the course of diagnostic work-up and treatment, there are many steps and options that may be available prior to going to IVF. Once couples have exhausted less invasive options and arrive at the point of needing IVF, the physical and psychological stressors become greater as compared with those whose infertility that can be addressed without the use of this advanced technology. As additional stressors are driving medical travel among couples engaging in cross-border reproductive travel, there would be an even greater need and benefit from support and counseling in this particular population. Given these findings, one wonders whether fertility clinics are doing their patients a disservice by tending exclusively to the medical aspects of treatment while disregarding the psychological aspects. Tending to patients through psychological support is not only the humane thing to do, it can also improve outcomes.

THE ROLE OF FACILITATORS OR REPRODUCTIVE TRAVEL BROKERS

Two studies—one in Australia on the home country end, and another in the Czech Republic at the receiving country end—took a closer look at the role of facilitators, also known as reproductive travel brokers. In Australia, access to IVF is relatively liberal, with no restrictions based on age or number of cycles, and significant subsidies to help support those pursuing it through their publicly funded healthcare system. Thus, the main reason Australians go overseas for cross-border reproductive travel is for egg donation or surrogacy mainly because access to either within Australia is strictly regulated and only allowed on an altruistic basis where the only expenses allowed to be reimbursed are those related to the actual medical costs. Going abroad to countries such as the United States, Greece, Spain, and South Africa gives Australians a wider range of choices, and ones that are much more quickly available than in their home country. Due to the accessibility of IVF in Australia, the facilitators were not typically working for those who were doing IVF without the addition of gamete donation or surrogacy (Millbank, p. 63).

Australian law professor Jenni Millbank conducted a study of facilitators of cross-border reproductive travel which found that the facilitators tout the benefits of reproductive travel without discussing much the risks (namely legal liabilities), oversight of quality assurance, emergency contingency plans, or financial ties. Researchers count facilitators as businesses within a subset of travel. Facilitators include both logistical and emotional support as part and parcel of their services. Millbank noted that facilitators emphasized the emotional aspects of the relationship in nurturing and care of the client, while downplaying the business aspect of the arrangement (Millbank).

Similarly, in her work on IVF brokers, Amy Speier found that the brokers used their friendly and empathetic personalities to provide support to their reproductive travelers and foster an open and trusting relationship with them. Through this support, the facilitators could be a source of familiarity and comfort to a couple undergoing reproductive travel (Speier 2011; 2016; Vindrola-Padros, 2019, pp. 118–119).

Speier found that IVF brokers are aware of the physical and emotional stress of undergoing IVF, and also of patients' feeling of not being cared for within the North American IVF system. They then jump in to fill this gap in care, addressing this important need in addition to the ones that are more tangible and quantifiable through a financial transaction. The brokers' website hones in on this desire to have one's emotions tended to, and this claim is bolstered by patient testimonials included on the brokers' websites (Speier, p. 45). In the context of the added stress and hope for infertility treatments, the care aspect of IVF overseas is also touted by the IVF brokers who are both aware of how important the affective nature of the relationship is, and also running a business with a goal to satisfy their patients. Congeniality and empathy are critical qualities for IVF brokers who often serve as the primary source of contact when the clients are in their home countries. Patients often chose an IVF broker based on the sense of "connection" they felt with them, and reviews refer to the "Czech family" abroad who helped look after them—both terms that highlight the affective relationship between the clients and the IVF brokers (Speier, pp. 60–61). Brokers perform labor-intensive work requiring availability at all hours of the day as they continue to guide and protect their clients as they travel overseas for their care. This intimate relationship is quite different from the experience of feeling like a number in an IVF mill at a clinic back at home (Speier, p. 77). Overall, through their own experiences with infertility and fertility treatments, the IVF brokers helped the patients feel calm, allayed their fears and helped coordinate all the details of their cross-border reproductive care.

In the Australian study, nearly half of the facilitators were lawyers, a third were general brokers, and the remaining fifth were medical professionals (Millbank, p. 63). One crucial profession that was not found among the Australian facilitators was mental health professionals or support counselors. This could be in keeping with Paula England's insight into the devaluation of care work and the lower pay for work traditionally carried out by women, underestimating the contribution of the work women do to organizational goals including profits. Further, adding insult to injury is using the altruistic motivations of care workers—the genuine desire for their patient to do well—as an excuse to pay them less (England, p. 382; 389). By extension, the lack of training required for the important work psychological counselors can do in the face of uncertainty and emotional stress as a couple travels abroad as part of their fertility journey devalues the importance of this work. Similarly, the underestimation of the benefit of psychological support in the success of reproductive treatment outcomes devalues both its necessity and potential to improve outcomes.

All the facilitators reported seeking out overseas clinicians who were trustworthy and competent, a judgment based on repeat reciprocal business. Of the eleven lawyers, there was a wide range of the divide between their role as facilitator versus lawyer—five provided independent legal counsel in the area of law, a couple of lawyers jointly practiced the legal services required for cross-border reproductive care while concurrently brokering reproductive transactions, while a couple acted as reproductive brokers while having to refer to lawyers specializing in reproductive law due to their expertise being in a different jurisdiction (Millbank, p. 63).

Facilitators marketed themselves not only as specialists and quality control supervisors, but also especially for their support services, something valuable and unique and not provided by typical clinical services. Quality control was typically not referred to by formal accreditation or any objective measure of success, but rather personal experience with a facility. While some of the facilitators noted they only worked with clinicians adhering to the society guidelines of the country they were practicing in, none of them knew how those guidelines compared with the more restrictive requirements in Australia. Reasons a facilitator stopped working with a given doctor included learning that they had mistreated an egg donor or posed unnecessary medical risk to a donor (via ovarian hyperstimulation) or recipient (transferring too many embryos). The facilitators stressed their role in relational support, taking care of both clients and reproductive donors, acting as infertility counselor, and protecting their patients from those who might take advantage of them; they often emphasized not being motivated by money (Millbank, pp. 64–65).

In an attempt to sort out ethical duties and limits to what they found acceptable, researchers asked facilitators if they had ever turned down a client or if they felt greater regulation was needed of the industry. While facilitators denied bad or unethical outcomes for any of their clients, many of them had horror stories of deals brokered by other facilitators. At the same time, they did not feel that additional oversight of the industry was warranted. In terms of conflict of interest, many of the heterogeneous facilitators felt there was a conflict of interest when one person performed several different roles, for example, lawyers also acting as facilitators. In contrast, none of the lawyers saw filling more than one role as a conflict of interest, but rather an extension of the services they were offering. They felt the dual coverage of services was driven by their clients, who often wanted considerable time for insight from the lawyer's past experiences with cross-border reproductive services, including but not limited to their legal services. Three of the lawyers did separate out their facilitation services by creating a separate agency sometimes under their spouse's name, in a tacit nod to the possibility of conflicts of interest. They would, however, often cross-refer between their agencies due to the specialized services each could offer. They did not discuss how being involved with both might bias the recommendations they were giving (Millbank, p. 66). Regardless, clearly one overarching group providing these various services and cross-referring to one another creates a conflict of interest that seems insurmountable without splitting up and maintaining separate the providers and owners of each needed service. Another concern is that a person attempting to provide multiple services may not have the adequate training and time to properly address the various services they are offering.

For the facilitators who were being paid by the overseas reproductive centers, their conflicts of interest were even more overt, as they were employees of or sponsored by certain center(s), while at the same time purportedly fulfilling their duties to advocate for and protect their clients. They still saw themselves as advocates for the clients. In contrast, the facilitators directly pairing parents with reproductive donors were more cognizant of the conflict, noting that while the prospective parents were their primary customer, they still cared about and protected reproductive donors, with one even saying the latter was their priority. All of the brokers used word of mouth to recruit new donors and saw them as a valuable resource they needed to shield. The facilitators provided separate and specialized support services to both intended parents and the reproductive donors, with trained counselors for the recipients and support staff for the donors (Millbank, p. 67).

Ethical considerations which came up in discussions with the facilitators include advertising for donation in low-income areas, paying too much thereby causing undue economic influence, using the same donor several times, transferring more than two embryos or not reimbursing clients when donors reneged. One facilitator noted that it was unethical to have a couple undergo multiple rounds of IVF knowing the likelihood of success was low, instead of referring them on for egg donation or surrogacy. Another facilitator thought it was unethical for Australian clinics to use Australian laws as a basis for refusal of transferring a patient's gametes or embryos overseas when they knew it was going to be used with egg donation or surrogacy in a country that permitted the practices. Presumably they felt the gametes belonged to the patient who should be able to do what they wanted with them, so long as the assisted reproductive technology was legal in the country it was being used, even if it was not legal in the country the patient was coming from. Interestingly enough, none of the facilitators felt the need for external regulation, though a minority did think peer-reviewed guidelines for standards would be helpful, and another minority of facilitators already reported adhering to U.S.-based industry code for surrogacy and egg donation. Some facilitators felt removing Australian regulations banning surrogacy and egg donation would actually better regulate the industry and keep things more ethical. One argued for the need for accreditation in this field, to prevent overcharging and incompetence (Millbank, pp. 69–70). Beyond those factors, accreditation would help ensure a minimum amount of education and training in the medical, psychological, financial, and legal aspects of care needed to be a good facilitator.

Recommendations for Standardization of Care, Challenges, and Goals for the Future

Overall, there are often additional social and/or religious factors beyond routine financial reasons for medical travel which can make reproductive travel more onerous. That, combined with the increased emotional and psychological stressors encountered by infertile couples, further compounded by those undergoing IVF overseas, leads to an even greater need for psychological support for patients participating in cross-border reproductive care. One provider currently fulfilling this need is the facilitator. However, in order to do it well, there should be a training and accreditation process required to work as a facilitator. That would augment the emotional support and counselor role many of the facilitators already provide and ensure that this support meets a standard of care. This could further be officialized by including it as a mandatory component of society guidelines regarding cross-border reproductive care. However, additional evaluation of the facilitator role including review of the European Society of Human Reproduction and Embryology (ESHRE)'s Good Practice Recommendations raises concerns about a conflict of interest and suggests the need to do away with the role of the medical reproductive broker while maintaining access to the variety of services they provide.

Given that use of reproductive technologies and gamete donation overseas has increased psychosocial stressors for the patients seeking out the care, there needs to be better guidance at both the medical and psychological levels. However, cross-border reproductive travelers often report difficulties and negative reactions when they seek medical advice regarding their plans in their home countries. Further, there is little practice guidance for counselors helping care for the reproductive travelers as well (Whittaker et al., p. 1675).

As for regulation issues in reproductive travel, home and host countries need to regulate cross-border assisted reproductive technologies on medical, legal, financial, psychological, and logistical bases. Three approaches are prohibition of cross-border reproductive travel, harmonization by equalizing regulations across borders, or harm-minimization by allowing it within specific safeguards. Harmonization is difficult as it requires uniformity in regulations across trading blocs. Harms can be minimized through unilateral regulation of travel networks and referral centers for clients with oversight of client, those providing gametes, with codes of practice and guidelines. There is also a need for cooperation between countries and hospitals in professional and hospital credentialing along with tracking outcomes data (Whittaker et al., p. 1680).

Given their overlapping geographic, governmental, and financial systems, one area where cross-border reproductive travel is easier to examine is within Europe. To this end, ESHRE's Good Practice Recommendations help guide practitioners and centers providing reproductive services to foreign patients. These recommendations touch upon four key areas: Equity, Quality, Safety; Evidence-based care (this second one is the largest category); Patient involvement; and Redress. For patient involvement, references to counseling and psychological support provided to the patient in their native language, and patients should be requested to bring the relevant details of prior work-up and treatment, especially in cases where there is not direct communication between local and overseas clinic (Shenfield et al., ESHRE).

Practical ways to apply ESHRE guidelines for cross-border reproductive care include ensuring reproductive travelers have informed consent with IVF, including the risks of ovarian hyperstimulation syndrome and death, having a registry of gamete donors to track repeat donors, an emphasis on single embryo transfers as a way to decrease the risks to mother and fetus that come with multiple gestation, and cutting out the middle man between gamete donors and the client in order to decrease the risk of exploitation (Shenfield et al., ESHRE). One classic example of this was one in which Romanian oocyte donors received $250 while the clinic received $11,000–$13,000 with the clinic pocketing the difference as profit (Whittaker et al., p. 1679).

Current implementation of ESHRE's Good Practice Recommendations is voluntary, via goodwill of participating institutions, promoted by encouraging as many professional societies to commit to adhering to the recommendations (ESHRE and Shenfield). Similarly, other authors note pan-European legislation is unlikely to be forthcoming any time soon, and in the interim, suggest clinics voluntarily adhere to minimum standards of care in the interest of transparency and responsibility (Thorn, Wischmann, and Blyth). The Good Practice Recommendations also discourage multiple order pregnancies and seeking a service abroad that is illegal in the native country, while encouraging access to full records, responsible referrals to quality sites abroad, counseling and psychological support in the native language, availability of redress via an ombudsman when things do not go as expected abroad. They also discourage fee splitting (clinic gets a portion of the fee of the clinic referred to) as an unethical practice. Further, they note that brokerage risks disrepute of the profession and also disproportionate enticement subjugating the needs and protection of the donor to those of the client/patient (p. 661).

On the one hand, there is the need to protect the donor in addition to advancing the needs of the recipient who is the client in the home country, a duty currently ascribed to the facilitator but perhaps not able to be fulfilled by them due to the inherent conflict of interest. On the other hand, there is the need for the psychological support currently provided by facilitators and needed especially not only for travelers going abroad but also especially those going abroad for reproductive treatments. How do we reconcile these two needs—one supposedly and the other more convincingly—addressed by the facilitator? One way to do this would be to separate these two essential roles served by the facilitator into two or more different roles. At present, a facilitator currently serves as the bridge between the donor and the recipient. However, just as a plaintiff and defendant should not be represented by the same lawyer, one should have serious doubts about a facilitator or medical travel broker's ability to serve both sides equally and impartially. Even if we separate out the roles of those whose primary duty is to the donor and those who serve the recipient, the risk remains of the two parties colluding in ways are unacceptable. The next question that arises is whether the same person brokering the deal should serve as the primary source of psychological support to the reproductive traveler(s). Due to a conflict of interest in serving both sides, these services should be separate. Also, the very idea of a "deal" to broker is one driven by prioritizing financial motives over meeting the medical and psychological needs of the key players involved in the equation. On this basis, I would argue that the role of a facilitator or medical reproductive broker as currently defined is indeed unethical.

In order to move things forward in a nod to the essential services provided by the broker, one could require a separation of services in two ways: the intended recipient of a given service, and the specific nature of the service. For example, those serving recipients/clients of cross-border reproductive services cannot be the same as those serving the donors. As for the specific nature of the service, those providing medical, legal, financial, and psychological support should have well-defined roles without one person's services reportedly spanning across multiple fields which would be a near impossibility to do well and without a conflict of interest. Accreditation should be required in each of these fields utilized in cross-border reproductive travel. Given the additional stressors not only of traveling abroad for healthcare, but also of dealing with infertility, psychological support should be a key component of the cross-border reproductive travelers' care, and should be provided by those with some form of training in the field whether done in the home or host country in the patient's native language.

Finally, if we say that the current role of the facilitator or reproductive travel broker is unethical and should be abolished, we still need to create a way to connect patients at home with their reproductive facility +/- donor overseas (if using sperm or egg donors) and to maintain some level of quality control. This should not be done as it often currently is based simply on one person's experience with a facility abroad. A more objective way to oversee quality control could be done by maintaining a database reflecting quality, outcomes, and complications data readily accessible to the public. This information should be available not only for the recipients or prospective clients from the home country, but also for the prospective donors from their respective countries. The data should be maintained by an oversight organization such as ESHRE. While adherence to the recommended Good Practice Recommendation guidelines is voluntary, the ability to be listed on such a database would be limited to those willing to provide that data. Or, at a minimum, it should be a red flag for a facility to be listed in the database but not provide their data. Another role that automatically arises by virtue of such a model would be that of a person well-versed in statistics reviewing the data supplied by overseas IVF centers for accuracy. The logistics of doing so are a whole other matter.

For now, a good place to start includes requiring a separation between those serving the recipient versus donor of reproductive services and passing legislation banning "brokers" from filling both roles; requiring a separation of the key players (medical, legal, financial, and psychological) in cross-border reproductive travel and banning one provider from double-dipping or self-referring, even if to a co-owned company by a different name, and abolishing the facilitator or reproductive travel broker. At the same time, there would still be a need for a coordinator role as well as a more objective means to connect the client or reproductive recipient with the institutions +/- the reproductive donor (if latter required) abroad. It is hopeful that attention to these aspects of cross-border reproductive care can help protect both the patient and the donor while maintaining a certain level of quality control.

ACKNOWLEDGMENT

The author would like to thank Professor Arthur Kuflik for his helpful comments on earlier drafts of this chapter.

REFERENCES

Bhatia, Rajani. 2014. "Cross-border sex selection: Ethical challenges posed by a globalizing practice." *International Journal of Feminist Approaches to Bioethics* 7(2): 185–193.

Cousineau TM, Domar AD. 2007. "Psychological impact of infertility." *Best Practice and Research Clinical Obstetrics and Gynecology* 29(2): 293–308.

Crozier GKD, Baylis F. 2010. "The ethical physician encounters international medical travel." *Journal of Medical Ethics* 36: 297–301.

Hanefeld J, Lunt N, Smith R, Horsfall D. 2015. "Why do medical travelers travel where they do? The role of networks in determining medical travel." *Social Science and Medicine* 124: 356–363.

Hudson N, Culley L, Blyth E, Norton W, Pacey A, Rapport F. 2016. "Cross-border assisted reproduction: A qualitative account of UK traveller's experiences." *Human Fertility* 19(2): 102–110.

Hughes EG, DeJean D. 2010. "Cross-border fertility services in North America: A survey of Canadian and American providers." *Fertility and Sterility* 94(1): e16–e19.

Jaspal R, Prior T, Denton J, Salim R, Banerjee J, Lees C. 2019. "The impact of cross-border IVF on maternal and neonatal outcomes in multiple pregnancies: Experience from a UK fetal medicine service." *European Journal of Obstetrics & Gynecology and Reproductive Biology* 238: 63–67.

Kjaer T, Albieri V, Jensen A, Kjaer SK, Johansen C, Dalton SO. 2014. "Divorce or end of cohabitation among Danish women evaluated for fertility problems." *Acta Obstetrica and Gynecologica Scandinavica* 93: 269–276.

Klonoff-Cohen H, Natarajan L. 2004. "The concerns during assisted reproductive technologies scale and pregnancy outcomes." *Fertility and Sterility* 81(4): 982–988.

Klonoff-Cohen H, Natarajan L, Klonoff E. "Validation of a New Scale Measuring Concerns of Women Undergoing Assisted Reproductive Technologies (CART)." *Journal of Health Psychology* 12(2): 352–356.

Malina A, Pooley JA. 2017. "Psychological consequences of IVF fertilization—Review of research." *Annals of Environmental and Agricultural Medicine* 24(4): 554–558.

Millbank J. 2018. "The role of professional facilitators in cross-border assisted reproduction." *Reproductive Biomedicine and Society Online* 6: 60–71.

Shenfield F et al. 2010. "Cross border reproductive care in six European countries." *Human reproduction* 25(6): 1361–1368.

Shenfield F. 2011. "Implementing a good practice guide for CRBC: Perspectives from the ESHRE Cross-Border Reproductive Care Taskforce." *Reproductive Biomedicine Online* 23: 657–664.

Thorn P, Wischmann T, Blyth E. 2012. "Cross-border reproductive services—suggestions for ethically-based minimum standards of care in Europe." *Journal of Psychosomatic Obstetrics & Gynecology* 33(1): 1–6.

Speier, A. 2011. "Brokers, consumers and the internet: How North American consumers navigate their infertility journeys." *Reproductive Biomedicine Online* 23(5): 592–599.

Speier, A. 2016. *Fertility holidays: IVF tourism and the reproduction of whiteness.* New York University Press: New York, NY.

Vindrola-Padros, C. 2020. Affective journeys in the imagination. In *Critical ethnographic perspectives on medical travel* (pp. 113–122). Routledge: New York, NY.

Waller KA, Dickinson JE, Hart RJ. 2017. "The contribution of multiple pregnancies from overseas fertility treatment to obstetric services in a Western Australia obstetric hospital." *Australian and New Zealand Journal of Obstetrics and Gynaecology* 57: 401–404.

Whittaker A, Inhorn MC, Shenfield F. "Globalised quests for assisted conception: Reproductive travel for infertility and involuntary childlessness." *Global Public Health* 14(12): 1669–1688.

Chapter 8

Complexity and Contradiction

Intimacy, Testimony, and Care in Humanitarian Aid

Elizabeth Lanphier

This chapter explores the affective experiences of those who travel in order to provide care, rather than to receive it. Humanitarian aid workers travel to, and then away from, the population for whom they are caring. By analyzing first-person accounts of humanitarian aid workers told in published memoir form, this chapter identifies three overlapping themes that strain and complicate emotional experiences of those traveling to provide humanitarian assistance abroad. One, is the forms of intimacy that aid workers are both drawn to and away from through international aid travel, exacerbated by their temporal-spatial transiency, cultural and linguistic differences among colleagues and beneficiaries, and the porosity between personal and professional boundaries. Two, is the role of advocacy and testimony on behalf of those to whom they are providing humanitarian assistance, and the ways in which this testimony wavers between a distanced, abstracted humanitarian ideal to help generalized others, and interpersonal, intimate, emotionally laden desire to help particular others. Three, intimacy and testimony relate not only to each other, but to a broader framework of care under which the humanitarian aid worker operates. The nature and role of care is at once abstracted and intimate, professional and personal, proximate and distant—distancing from one's traditional caring relationships at home is necessary to care for distant others to whom one becomes proximate through travel. Care can be an act, an approach, or an affect—and though it can be all of these at once, affection need not necessarily translate into action, and action does not always or even often entail affection.

For the purposes of this chapter, "humanitarian aid" refers to foreign assistance carried out by independent non-governmental organizations

(NGOs) or supra-governmental organizations, such as the United Nations (UN) and its various agencies. "Humanitarian worker" or "aid worker" indicates foreigners or expatriates ("expats") who are deployed on a temporary assignment or "mission" to a "field" location, which means outside of their country of origin or primary country of residence. The "field" can be any setting in which a humanitarian project is carried out, though those working in "the field" may frequently draw further distinctions between work conducted in a country's capital or centralized office, and regional "field" offices that are in more remote locations and often closer to beneficiary populations.

Most international humanitarian agencies also employ "local" or "national" staff depending on the preferred terminology of the agency. These are citizens/residents of the country in which aid is being provided. There are significant political, economic, cultural, and equity issues wrapped up within the national/international staff divide that cannot be adequately explored in this chapter. Importantly, national staff often constitute a robust portion of project staffing, supply local knowledge and consistency despite rotating international staff, and often remain in subordinate roles to international staff despite their local expertise and constancy. Depending on the agency, local staff may or may not be able to attain leadership roles within a given humanitarian organization. While systemic racism, colonial histories, and white and Western supremacy are critiques directed at international humanitarianism for some time, there is a renewed awareness of these deep-rooted concerns in light of global contemporary support for, and mobilization behind, the Black Lives Matter movement.

As an example, Doctors Without Borders/Medecins Sans Frontieres (MSF), a medical humanitarian organization that has headquarters offices in Europe, North America, and Australia, and carries out field work in response to conflict, natural disaster, and medical emergency around the world, responded to an open letter signed by more than 1,000 current and former staff members calling on the organization to address racist and white supremacist practices. In response, MSF leadership noted its intent to seriously restructure its organization, with particular attention to "breaking the glass ceiling for locally hired staff"; revising disparate compensation schemes (in which international staff make higher salaries and per diem); levels of risks staff are exposed to (e.g., only international staff, not locally hired staff, are generally guaranteed evacuation from unsafe situations); and reviewing "medical double standards" and "broader issues of harassment, abuse and discrimination" (MSF 2020). Some of this work, if undertaken carefully and successfully, may address many of the internal tensions and contradictions that this chapter raises with regards to intimacy, testimony, and care, across cultural and racial divides in humanitarian settings. Such efforts are unlikely, however, to radically overhaul the fact of global humanitarian aid, or the emotional and affective challenges internal to it.

As Emily Bauman recently argued, "[m]emoir has for some time played a significant role in the expansion and interpretation of the humanitarian industry," including "Henri Dunant's 1862 memoir *A Memory of Solferino*" that instigated the establishment of global humanitarianism in the form of the "ICRC (International Committee of the Red Cross) and Geneva Convention, and Moritz Thomsen's 1969 memoir *Living Poor: A Peace Corps Chronicle* that helped promote participation in the US Peace Corps" (Bauman 2019, 83). Bauman describes the genre of the memoir as an effective "ambassador" of experience "from the field to the larger public, orientated as it is to personal experience and testimony" (2019, 83). With its orientation to "personal experience and testimony," memoir as a literary form is both an instantiation and site of further reflection on the nature of personal experience and testimony, which contribute to the form and function of humanitarian aid. The genre of the humanitarian memoir is relatively novel: Bauman notes most humanitarian memoirs have been published in the twenty-first century, but the growing literary field can already be classified in subgenres (85). Bauman takes up the subgenre of the humanitarian "founder" memoir, "because there is more at stake in their [founders'] need to legitimise the organisation whose founding they describe" and Bauman's target of study is a narrative analysis of "humanitarian ideology" (86). I instead analyze the subgenre of humanitarian participant memoir. Bauman describes participant stories as "coming-of-age" or "rites of passage" narratives (85) that follow an arc from innocent naivete and idealism, to critical cynicism about humanitarian aid, to a renewed affirmation of values achieved through a more thorough understanding and experience of the work.

The published humanitarian memoir is a growing literary genre, and I have focused on a narrative analysis of several particular humanitarian protagonists. I have chosen these texts because they are in first-person memoir form, and are specifically about the writers' humanitarian work-life experience (rather than featuring only the personal or professional aspects of humanitarian work, or biography that offers a third-person account of humanitarian worker experience). I have specifically selected memoirs that cover an extended period of time, and work across various NGOs, in order to analyze evolutions in the affective experiences of the authors across time, place, and role, to get at a core of affective experience related to the structure of humanitarian work, rather than reflect a specific time and place of humanitarian engagement. Close reading these texts affords concrete examples of the complexities and contradictions inherent in intimacy, testimony, and care within international humanitarian work. Three of the memoirists are non-clinical humanitarian workers, Jessica Alexander, Kenneth Cain, and Heidi Postlewait, all of whom work in coordinator roles for international humanitarian agencies, interfacing with medical relief operations. Alexander and Postlewait both recount formative experiences of encountering beneficiaries with medical needs in clinical settings. The final memoirist analyzed in this chapter is physician and surgeon Andrew Thomson, whose work goes from providing medical aid to restore the sick and injured to life, to forensically examining the dead in Rwanda and Bosnia, two sites of genocidal atrocity. These selected memoirs are not meant to encompass the experience of all humanitarian aid workers, nor the entire genre of the humanitarian memoir. However, they exemplify patterns arising in humanitarian aid, in which one travels far from their location of origin to provide care to distant others, regarding intimacy, testimony, and care. These patterns include the dance of detachment and dissociation with intimacy and advocacy, that comprise the complicated ethical and emotional experience of humanitarian care, which is always both done at a distance from one's starting point (geographically, but also often emotionally and psychologically), yet also intimately and immediately with colleagues and beneficiaries in the setting of a humanitarian intervention.

A goal of humanitarian relief is not only to travel abroad to attend to the immediate suffering of beneficiaries—that is, to go elsewhere to provide necessary care, but to bear witness to their plight in order to return from abroad able to advocate effectively for improved conditions, necessary resources, and political change. Functioning in high-stakes humanitarian situations may involve the closing off of emotion: dissociation from human response, ironically, in the name of humanitarian response. This happens in part through the physical distancing of humanitarian care: it is something done "over there," in the field, abroad, far away. At the same time, humanitarianism is motivated by the idea of shared humanity, and the beauty and dignity of the whole person, a beauty and dignity that hopefully the provider of humanitarian care carries with her in her work, and upon her return, as a witness and advocate. In the end, both practitioner and patient risk being rendered less than human: the practitioner is encouraged, or even supported, to distance her own emotions from the intervention as a mode of coping; the humanity of the beneficiary, which drives the objectives and rationale of humanitarian response, is often minimized in order to achieve necessary emotional dissociation by the provider navigating a stressful and traumatic humanitarian crisis, or by being rendered a data point, a piece of epidemiological or political data, a "beneficiary" rather than a human.

Although it raises complexities and contradictions intrinsic in the emotional experiences of caring for others in humanitarian contexts, this chapter concludes on a note of productive tension between detachment and distance, intimacy and affection. The emotional dance of care contributes to its strength and urgency. As theorized within feminist ethics and the ethics of care, care itself can be many things: personal, political, professional, intimate, distanced, affectionate, aloof. Virginia Held (2006) understands care as a relational activity that is both a practice and a value. Nel Noddings (1984) has analyzed the affective experience of, and relations involved in, caring as kind of moral exchange between the one-caring and the cared-for. Noddings takes a broad view of what care is, yet locates is mainly within families and homes. Joan Tronto (2006) and Sarah Ruddick (1998) both acknowledge care is a form of work, in addition to a relationship, whether or not this work is formally recognized and compensated. Noddings along with Carol Gilligan center the affective components of caring relationships, whereas others such as Diemut Bubeck (1995) take up the functional rather than the emotional role of care. Peta Bowden (1997) does not require that care be a specific kind of affective or functional relationship, and instead conceptualizes care as the practice of valuing others.

Joan Tronto and Bernice Fisher develop care outside of interpersonal relationships and into public and political ones. They describe care as an "activity that includes everything that we do to maintain, continue, and repair 'our world' so that we can live in it as well as possible." Such activity expands far beyond the family or home, to include "a variety of social, economic, and political institutions" (as quote in Brandsen 2006, 206). My own work theorizes care as an institutional practice, in addition to an interpersonal one, in which we have obligations as participants in social structures to support the needs of others with whom we participate in said structures, including obligations to unknown others, through care practices (Lanphier 2021). Rather than pitting care against justice orientations, as care ethics sometimes appears to, I construe care as a necessary element of justice, and justice as necessary to care, a concept I call "care justice" (Lanphier 2021). A unifying feature of care, across these different theories and perspectives, is that care is always an exchange, between the cared-for and the caring-one (whether these roles are filled by specific individuals, types of individuals, or communities and institutions). This exchange is itself an opportunity for arriving anew at emotional encounters with others, and with the self.

THE HUMANITARIANS

Jessica Alexander calls her 2013 memoir *Chasing Chaos: My Decade in and out of Humanitarian Aid*. In it, she chronicles her draw to the international humanitarian sector, propelled there by loss and grief at home: her mother died when Alexander was twenty-two years old and Alexander says, "if I could die at age fifty [like her mother], I wanted a more meaningful profession" than her job working for advertising agencies in New York City (2013,

16). She traveled to Central America as a tourist where she encountered expat foreign aid workers. There she "saw something out there far bigger than my own New York existence," and "wanted to be part of it," so Alexander "returned home determined to pursue aid work" (17). Her motives are in part to participate in something bigger than herself and effect change, to live a life she imagined "would be filled with adventure and rewarding, intellectually intriguing work" (17). Yet she acknowledges that she also "*was* looking for a way to dodge the painful repercussions of my mom's death" and be "distracted" from the "grief that still lingered" (17). As she says: "there was other suffering out in the world, and I wanted to touch it" (17). She admits that at the time of writing her memoir, reflecting on a decade of doing the work, it remains hard "to distill my feelings into a single, succinct motive" that led her into humanitarian aid (17).

Though her motives were muddled, she approached humanitarian work with a quick-learned savvy, realizing that she would need appropriate credentials in order to pursue the increasingly professionalizing and competitive arena of international humanitarian work. Alexander enrolls in graduate school to earn multiple masters degrees, and takes on field work initially as an intern during graduate school in Mozambique and Rwanda, and then through multi-month postings in conflict and disaster zones including Darfur during the height of conflict and internal displacement, and Sri Lanka and Indonesia following the 2004 tsunami in South East Asia.

Alexander's experience in the field takes off at the same time three humanitarian workers from an earlier generation publish their co-authored memoir *Emergency Sex and Other Desperate Measures* (2004). The book recounts first-person entries from Heidi Postlewait, a New York City social worker turned UN secretary and then field personnel; Kenneth Cain, a Harvard Law graduate looking to do different work than his fellow graduates, who gets involved with human rights law; and Andrew Thomson, an Australian physician and surgeon who left a career in academic medicine to care for patients in conflict zones.

Thomson's background training and experience prepared him for the technical contributions he would make to field work as a medical doctor. However, both Postlewait and Cain, despite their educations in the United States, were relatively unprepared for the fieldwork on which they embarked. Writing about the role of the personal in the professional in 2012, Anne-Meike Fechter notes a trend toward "the professionalization of relief and development work," and suggests that this move toward professionalization has not helped better recognize the role of the personal in aid work, as much as it has "contributed to relegating it further into the background" (2012, 1391). Postlewait, Cain, and Thomson all met in Cambodia in 1993, the first international postings for Postlewait and Cain, but not for Thomson.

Postlewait and Cain begin their humanitarian careers when it was still possible to enter into field work with more good intention than good experience. They then cut their teeth on postings in Somalia and Rwanda in the mid-1990s, crises that defined and directed the future of humanitarian aid and humanitarian professionalization.

INTIMACY

International aid work dances between the personal and professional. Fechter suggests that the very phenomenon of aid worker memoirs and blogs demonstrates the "ways in which the personal and professional are intertwined in aid work" (1388). Yet Fechter also underscores a reluctance to acknowledge the personal dimensions of aid work, due to what she argues is a set of idealized commitments to selflessness or altruism. Alexander, Postlewait, Cain, and Thomson all illustrate versions of this vacillation between personal or instrumental objectives of their humanitarian careers, and putatively altruistic motives. Alexander acknowledges she was avoiding grief, yet also compelled to participate in something bigger than herself. Postlewait was energized by the social work she did in New York City, yet it was the dissolution of a marriage in which her altruistic principles were at odds with her husband's talent agent career, and the need to make a quick and sufficient income following her divorce, that spur her to work for the UN, rather than a sense of humanitarian spirit. After feeling he has failed at the work he set out to do in Haiti, Thomson retreats to UN headquarters doing medical exams for returning or deploying expats, an apparent recognition of his personal need for a hiatus from the stressors and trauma of intense field work, only to be driven back by the sense of mission into an even more grim context cataloging bodies massacred in Rwanda.

The selflessness might also be selfish: a personal need to play a martyr, or desire to be a savior. This is part of the complexity of the collapse of personal and professional into each other with humanitarian work: the personal and professional mutually compliment, and yet also contradict, each other. What looks initially like prioritizing a professional sense of duty to aid, to the detriment of interpersonal connection, may also be the very personal desire to distance oneself from intimacy, or to seek fulfillment in travel and adventure. Alexander abandons her fiancé for her aid work when her "twenty-five-year-old-self felt sure it wasn't possible to" pursue a humanitarian aid career "*and* be married at the same time." In breaking off her engagement, she says "it was the first time, but certainly not the last, that my personal life would take a backseat to this career" (46). Yet when she talks about the lack of connection she felt to her fiancé as her graduate studies progressed, it seems less clear that she traded intimate connection for her career as much as her career made plain the lack of intimacy in her romantic life.

Cain develops a fulfilling personal life in a romantic relationship with a French expat while working in a remote village in Haiti, but feels compelled to enlist for work in Rwanda to contribute to more urgent humanitarian response. He chooses tense, traumatic, and erratic work over the more controlled environment of his current deployment, and the intimacy and stability it affords in his romantic relationship. Assessing retention rates for international deployments within one MSF operational center, Korff and colleagues note that even as aid becomes better compensated and professionalized, it operates on a temporary mission model to retain the sense of volunteerism. Yet agencies anticipate re-deployment despite not offering long-term or permanent field contracts (Korff et al 2015) because it is assumed that aid workers hold altruistic values, exhibit flexibility in response time to emerging crises, and are willing to work in "dangerous locations" (Korff et al 2015, 523). These assumptions play out in Cain's decision to leave Haiti for Rwanda, to deploy to where he perceives there is more urgent work to be done.

There is a sense of both contingency and predictability, or predictability of contingency, with humanitarian work. Alexander learns that "keeping some degree of distance from the short-termers"—those working on weeks or month stints in a field context as opposed to months to years—"was how we dealt with the transience of this existence" (59). Connection needs to be measured carefully, knowing that while everyone is temporary, some are more so. Korff and colleagues note reports from the International Committee of the Red Cross (ICRC) and People in Aid demonstrating "difficulties in balancing private and professional life" and secondarily, "lack of career opportunities" as primary motivators for discontinuing aid work, while "negative attitudes such as disillusionment, frustration, or boredom . . . are only accountable for a small minority of job exits" from the international aid sector (2015, 526). This suggests that intimacy and care are central to aid worker experience—especially being alienated from existing intimate or caregiving relationships, obligations, or connections, while working abroad.

And yet plenty of intimacy occurs in humanitarian contexts. The very title *Emergency Sex* foregrounds the role of sex in the complicated professional/personal lives of humanitarian workers, especially when international staff often live together or live on the same compound in which they work, seeing their colleague in a towel in the morning before seeing them at the office during the day. Alexander describes frustration with the "lack of control over our most basic needs" while working abroad (4). On the one hand, aspects of daily living are taken care of for expats: housing is provided, furnished, and maintained for them; several or all meals a day are made by cooks; drivers provide all transport to and from work and anywhere else—often this is for safety as much as convenience. Yet this also limits freedoms to choose for oneself.

Sex is something over which an individual aid worker can take control for herself, including in order to relinquish control over to a sexual partner or to the sex itself. Though the taking and ceding of control is more complicated when the sex is between expatriates and local staff or residents due to underlying imbalances of power and control. The foreign aid worker might feel she has no control over her basic needs of daily living, but retains control to leave her assignment, to evacuate away from a crisis. This option is rarely available to local residents and locally hired staff. Fechter suggests that the role of the aid worker body, particularly with regards to intimacy and sex, is an underdeveloped area of inquiry, especially the ways in which aid workers are intertwined in either consensual or coerced sexual relationships with local staff or residents in the countries in which foreigners work as international aid actors. We might say that these international–local relationships can fall within a spectrum between consent and coercion, and sometimes in the realm of non-consent (Fyfe and Lanphier 2020) or quasi-consent (or coercion), given power disparities between foreign aid-providers and local beneficiaries or staff. Alexander recounts how one of her more experienced colleagues described humanitarian aid as a "take-it-or-leave-it relationship"—beneficiaries can either accept or reject aid as a whole package, usually with minimal input on its terms, method of delivery, or scope—and remarks "there's no situation where the power between two groups is more lopsided. Except . . . maybe prison" (365).

Cain, Postlewait, and Thomson (whose relationship with the fellow expat, Suzanne, in Rwanda motivates them to seek geographically proximate posts in Eastern Europe, and then in New York) each develop sustained physical and emotional connections while working in the field. Yet sexual encounters in field contexts are also just as or more often described as devoid of emotion. Sex can serve a perfunctory, physical purpose. Alexander recounts meeting a "hot Australian" at a party in Khartoum, the capital of Sudan, when she first deployed there. She was initially cautious about him, and did not see him again before traveling on to Darfur. But upon her return to Khartoum for a brief respite, she immediately reconnects with him and says, "it didn't even matter who he was. After so many long, hot days made worse by lonely nights, just touching another human being felt incredible. I had one night with him, and we stayed up until the sun rose, me savoring every affectionate hour" (181). The next day, when her flight is canceled and she can stay another day in the capital, the Australian discloses that his girlfriend from home is arriving this very day to visit. Alexander "realized that this was my first encounter with how hollow this work could make you—how easy it was to shirk attachments, when you are always leaving one place for another, and how hard it was to build anything resembling a sustainable relationship" (182). The intimacy of the sexual encounter in the field is also a form of distancing from intimate emotional relationships back home, and the connection to home is a barrier to deepening any intimacy in the field. Later in her time in Darfur Alexander meets "a German guy who was in town for a few weeks doing a water assessment. We had nothing in common. In fact I found him pretty annoying. But I hooked up with him anyway" (200). The physical intimacy was a way to "alleviate the boredom and the monotony of my nights" (200), says Alexander, but it was a form of limited intimacy, sex without real interest or connection.

Postlewait, who coins the term "emergency sex," has possibly the most fraught relationships with intimacy, and intimate relationships, of any of the memoirists surveyed here. She describes intense sexual and or romantic relationships with primarily Black men (Postlewait is a white American woman), who are often local to the places in which she is working. She has a multi-day affair with a Masai tribesman in Mombasa, Kenya, before deploying to Somalia. Postlewait notices as she walks with James, the Masai tribesman, "the other solitary white woman, all fairly young and attractive, with their own Masai tribesman" and remarks to herself "great, now I've turned into one of those rich white chicks who pick up poor, attractive men in third world countries for sex" (92). This self-awareness does not change her mind or her actions. When she understands that James is not allowed on the hotel premises where she is staying, she joins him in his village, where they smoke pot and talk about Bob Marley with his friends, and have sex around the clock for several days.

Between Postlewait and James there are exchanges of sex, intimacy, connection, care, but also money. When Postlewait is ready to resume her regularly scheduled life of expat hotels and humanitarian deployment, James accompanies her back by bus. She says she "wrestled with my thoughts the entire morning," wondering "what does he really expect from me? Is it possible that this man with the body of a warrior and the smile of Cupid who spends his days walking half-naked with the tourists on the beach, who didn't hesitate to approach me, could not be a prostitute? At what point is one considered a prostitute?" (100). Postlewait construes a false dichotomy between male and female sex workers, suggesting that it is clear when a "woman is costumed," and a man rolls up in a car, the woman "gets in, takes care of business, a monetary transaction follows. It's over for him. The woman doesn't expect—doesn't want—anything more than the cash" (100). Postlewait takes it a woman buying sex wants something else for her money, though she may just be referring to herself and her own needs for the transaction: "Why do we need to create the false sense of emotional ties?" Despite this emotional scaffolding she says she feels "guilty," like "I have used and kicked to the curb another human being" As they part ways she tells James she will write and "I hand him two hundred-dollar bills. He takes them, smiles, and walks away" (100). Her account is less a gendered preference for transactional sex as much as it reflects the internal contradiction of sexual intimacy in humanitarian settings. Moreover, transactional sexual relationships take nuanced forms, no matter the gender or sex identities of those involved, especially in settings with inherent power imbalances. In humanitarian contexts transactional sex can be implicit as much as explicit.

There is a desire for connection and closeness, yet also a holding at a distance: humanitarian workers are transient, impermanent, in motion. Postlewait could stay in a remote Masai village outside of Mombasa, but she won't. She intends to continue to move on to the next humanitarian emergency. Travel across new borders and to new crises is the one given in this particular form of travel-care work. Just as Alexander's sexual liaison with the Australian in Khartoum was circumscribed by her presumed temporariness in the capital, her relationship with a Rwandan man during a several month stint there was certain to conclude when her time was up. Cain's relationship to the Frenchwoman Genevieve in Haiti was happy and connected, yet delimited by his next assignment and move—to Rwanda. Postlewait describes a series of relationships with local men in subsequent assignments: with Yusuf, a Somali interpreter with a wife back in Toronto, while stationed in Mogadishu, and with Marc, a Haitian man in Port-au-Prince with whom she lived for three years and started a business, until his sudden death. Only Thomson, who shares little about sexual relationships during his humanitarian work, concludes his story in a romantic partnership: he and Suzanne remain together in New York City, and plan to build a home in Cambodia.

Postlewait's relationship with Yusuf begins as "emergency sex." They had been connecting over time, though Yusuf's marriage had kept their flirtation from becoming sexual. One night they ate together at the mess hall and then walked back toward the living quarters when they spot a sniper and "we panic and start running nowhere and everywhere in circles" when "a passing UN soldier grabs" Postlewait, rolling her "to the ground and up against a building" while "Yusuf dives under a jeep stuck in the sand nearby. A round pings off the driver's door." After some time passes "Yusuf and I get up and run around to the safe side of the building. And then the strangest thing happens. I want to rip my clothes off, rip Yusuf's clothes off, and just fuck him right there" (132). This sex "has to be right now . . . Now. An emergency. Emergency sex." They start to resume their walk toward her room, but instead she pulls him into an empty tea shack where they have sex. As they "leave the tea shack, still clinging to each other" they pass a "dark lumpy form" and "Yusuf says matter-of-factly that it's a dead body" (132). Postlewait starts "sobbing" and "can't stop" (133). The intensity of fear, intimacy, connection, and death, are all wrapped together.

Alexander's encounter with the Australian is a form of emergency sex, an urgent need for intimate connection that also allows for a distancing from the harsh realities of difficult and demoralizing humanitarian care work. Cain describes his first experience in a conflict setting when he travels to Tel Aviv and connects with a friend of a friend, an Israeli woman who shows him a scud attack in the distance from her roof, after which they fall into a sexual encounter that reminds them "we are young and we are alive" (19). Emergency sex is both connection and distraction, it is a fantasy escape from the challenges and atrocities faced in humanitarian work, yet it is also a real and tangible connection with another body, and with the self. This is what makes the emergency sex form of intimacy involved in humanitarian care a constant tension: it is a way to embrace another, and emotional experience, while also a distancing from others and emotional experience—an escape from the self or from the context. Whether because of the sheer intensity of the situation, or also because of the geographical distance from one's "home" self, these encounters seem to describe experience unlike one's behaviors and practices "at home." Emergency sex happens "over there"—in the field, abroad.

While it is impossible to offer a full analysis of the added complexities when sexual encounters occur across cultural, racial, and economic difference in humanitarian settings, especially between so-called "expat" workers and local residents, the complex contradictions between intimacy and distancing, connection and transaction, already present *between* expatriates risk being all the more layered and complex between expatriates and local residents. This is not to suggest that there cannot be emotionally connected, mutual affection and collaboration by differently-situated individuals, there certainly can. Postlewait describes feeling at home in Haiti, and with Marc, a pride in Haiti's history that she wants to inhabit herself. Once she and Marc settle into their romantic partnership, she decides that "Haiti will be my home. I belong here" (227). Cain observed Postlewait as "genuinely in love this time with Marc the person—not a country and not a conflict, but with Marc" (232). Cain contrasts Marc with Yusuf, in whom he suggests Postlewait had a project or cause more than partner: "with [Yusuf] came a clan to adopt, a culture to learn, a wife to hate, a scandal to withstand" (232). As Cain characterizes it, Postlewait's relationship in Somalia was part of her commitment to the work and to the place—or as he says, the country and the conflict—in which she is working—not to the person.

Postlewait's own description suggests some part of being intimate with the country and its crises as integral to her interpersonal relationship: she wants Marc, but she also desires to be part of his country, to belong there and adopt it as her own. Perhaps this is due to an affiliative recognition of herself in and with Haiti, a country that fended off its colonial power to become and remain sovereign. Yet it also risks exerting an imperial power over Haiti, a desire for appropriation and colonization. These are only two, non-exhaustive, examples of inter-cultural relationships between expatriate aid workers and local residents where they work. Yet they show how intimacy, both emotional and sexual, but also the intimacy of care work, and the intimacy of living and working among and on behalf of others who are suffering, does not offer any simple or direct analysis, but is part of a layered and interwoven whole.

TESTIMONY

Jessica Alexander imagines explaining to friends and new acquaintances the work she does by saying "I make my living off the suffering of strangers" (255). She is far from the first to acknowledge that crises and human suffering are the very reasons humanitarian workers have jobs. Although international humanitarian workers are always merging the private and professional when they live and work together, share meals and trauma, bathrooms and bedrooms, the intimacy is also tempered by a distancing and emotional or psychic isolation, as already discussed. Alexander also reflects on a kind of "loneliness" twinned with an "unrelenting feeling of futility" because of the "endlessness to the crisis" that her efforts are responding to, and the inability of the aid work to which she has committed her personal and professional life to end the "real problems" facing the place and people she is there to support (5). There is an intimacy to the interactions humanitarian aid workers have with suffering, "suffering was all around me," Alexander writes, but "people coped" (256). To cope with the suffering is in part to recognize an intimacy with it, and to also distance oneself from the intimacy of it.

Bearing witness, or humanitarian testimony, is an implicit, and sometimes explicit, objective of humanitarian assistance. MSF centers bearing witness (or in French, *témoignage*) in its work, and as part of its founding charter (Lanphier 2018). Part of MSF's founding is indebted to doctors working with the ICRC during the Biafran war who were unwilling to accept the ICRC's interpretation of neutrality as negating publicly speaking out about atrocities witnessed in the field, and formed their own NGO (MSF) that was committed to neutrality and impartiality, but did not see these as inconsistent principles with advocacy and bearing witness (Lanphier 2018). Whether or not an individual aid worker speaks out publicly, or works for an agency with an overt commitment to testimony or advocacy, arguably any aid work directly in contact with beneficiaries bears witness to the suffering of others. And arguably to bear witness to suffering entails some form of testimony about what one witnesses, even if it is private testimony to the self.

"After months of weekly camp meetings" in an internally displaced person (IDP) camp in Darfur where Alexander worked, she says that "Ahmed, the camp committee leader, and I were friends" (189). Ahmed was a local Sudanese leader, with whom Alexander could only communicate through a translator, but she says they had "an unspoken understanding" (189). This is yet another form of intimacy and distance: understanding across cultural and language divide. She recounts how one day Ahmed asks her to come see his niece who is sick, and she reminds him that she is not a doctor, but he presses her for her help. Alexander describes seeing "his sister, meek and soft" on a floor with a "large pillow covered by a towel on her lap" and a "stoic and expressionless" face. When she "slowly pulled back the towel covering the pillow" Alexander could see her "tiny and frail" newborn, "her head twice its size, swollen and puffy. It looked like a balloon floating on top of a skeleton" (190).

After witnessing this scene that left her "queasy," having "never seen anything like this" Alexander immediately and unreflectively commits to transporting the baby to Khartoum for medical care (191). She acknowledges that her "personal relationship . . . with Ahmed" was part of what "jolted me into action" and the feeling that among so many humanitarian atrocities outside her control (attacks, rapes, and rains that flooded the IDP camp sewage and led several children to drown) this one sick child was something she "could actually do something about" (192). Bearing witness to so many crises without feeling capable of being able to change their course either demands or develops an attitude of detachment. Yet to translate that witnessing into advocacy allows for, and perhaps to be done effectively, requires, some intimacy of connection to the issue, if not also to those impacted by it.

The problem, of course, is that not all those impacted by a crisis are able to connect on an intimate register with those who could help them, and those who could help might resist connection knowing their ability to aid or rescue is limited. Initially, the only medical doctor available to consult is Alexander's father, living thousands of miles away in the United States, who diagnoses the infant as hydrocephalic based on her description. Her friendship with Ahmed brings her to the baby, her family connection to her father arrives at a diagnosis, and the certainty that without medical treatment the baby will die. Both connections are intimate, yet also at a distance. They also place Alexander in the unique position to advocate for this baby, to give testimony to her specific suffering.

When Alexander raises this baby's medical condition with her colleagues, however, she is met with inaction. She asks to put the baby and mom on a plane to Khartoum for transport to hospital, but is told that the World Food

Program (WFP) running planes between Darfur and Khartoum "won't let IDPs on the flights. You know that." When Alexander offers to pay the costs herself, she is told "we can't pick and choose IDPs to fly to Khartoum for medical treatment" (192) and that if Alexander pays directly it will still appear as though the agency supported the decision and its costs. Another colleague who coordinates health programs in the local clinic tells Alexander that they had other individuals who needed higher level health care in the IDP camps that they couldn't transport to Khartoum, either. When Alexander asks what happened to them, she learns "two of them have died already" (193).

Unlike the clinicians facing unmet medical need daily in the camp settings, Alexander says "I hadn't been confronted with this degree of clinical detachment before" and she couldn't imagine how she could "go back to Ahmed and tell him that there was nothing I could do, nothing that the humanitarian community could do, to help" (193). While Alexander advocated for the infant, and the role of humanitarian actors is to "save lives and reduce suffering," her colleagues point to the reality that "we can't save everyone" (194). She acknowledges that her "personal relationship with Ahmed was clearly blurring my logic" but also felt that the humanitarian response was below a basic standard of care, and not "the best we could do" (194). The dance of intimacy and detachment is also part of the dance of advocacy and testimony. It is intimacy of friendship, and first-hand witnessing of a particular individual's suffering, that moves her to advocate for this one child, but also to recast her understanding of sufficient aid response to all putative beneficiaries. Ultimately through a series of fortunate persuasions and circumstances Alexander gets Ahmed's niece and her baby on a plane to Khartoum and to the hospital—though the baby does not survive, even with hospitalization.

Postlewait also experiences the intimacy, and frustration, of a medical provider's clinical encounter, with a patient in Somalia. Postlewait meets an expatriate medical doctor, angry about "what they do to women here"— genital cutting—a fact to which Postlewait resists bearing witness because she says: "I like the Somalis, and I don't want to believe it" (175). The doctor invites Postlewait into the exam room to see a Somali woman's genitals herself, even though she serves no clinical purpose in the medical encounter. Postlewait describes the woman as having "no vulva. There's nothing there, it's all been sliced off and sewn shut. The doctors now have to reopen her so she can give birth to her child" (175).

The doctor apologizes to Postlewait, saying "I'm sorry . . . I had to share it with someone, a woman." Postlewait describes the doctor as looking "somehow fortified, like she passed her trauma on to me," but wonders "who do I share it with now?" (175). She goes on with her day preoccupied, wondering if the young woman who cleans her room, whom she befriended, has been "mutilated too" (177). She decides to ask Yusuf, the Somali man with whom she was involved, about it, but worried he might defend the practice of genital mutilation, and this would be a kind of testimony within their relationship, a disclosure from which they could not recover. Yusuf confirms that all Somali women are mutilated, but that he does not endorse the practice. He adds that in educated families "women only lose a small part of their vulva and are not sewn shut," as though, Postlewait remarks, "a small part of your vulva is a minor concession" (178). Here the transference of trauma takes hold in intimate testimony, to a colleague, with a partner. It also had likely no benefit to the Somali woman whose intimate clinical encounter was made public, her own privacy not protected for the benefit of external eyes that could do nothing to change her own circumstances.

Andrew Thomson is the one humanitarian across these memoirs who is a physician. A demoralizing experience of providing clinical care in Haiti compelled him to return to UN Headquarters in New York, where he was a physician examining expatriate staff pre or post deployment. Yet his sense of mission and purpose spur him to return to the field—where he works in Rwanda following the genocide. There he is not restoring the living, but cataloging the dead, forensically examining exhumed mass graves in order to prosecute genocidal perpetrators. Thomson describes the "shower that our engineer has rigged on-site" as the "best part of my day" when the "piping hot water under pressure" removes the "pieces of strangers' flesh and bone" that had been stuck to his hair and skin (237).

Thomson has moved from the intersubjectivity of clinical encounters, to the detachment of digging up graves. At the same time, this work draws him intimately close with the lives of others: the traumatic endings those lives met. He is inhabiting their bodies as they stick to his in an intimate exchange of flesh, quite differently than the intimacy of emergency sex or emotional connection among aid workers. Yet it is a kind of productive intimacy that allows him to fully bear witness, to offer literal testimony on behalf of countless unknown others. It is opposite the experience of Alexander, cognizant of the endlessness of crisis and the feeling of futility amidst massive unmet needs, who homes in on a particular intimate relationship, her friendship with Ahmed, that spurs her particular engagement in a specific act of rescue. Thomson's beneficiaries are all dead, there is no further futility, the crisis *has* ended. His advocacy and testimony, however, is part of all that can be done, to recognize the humanity of the dead, and to hold others accountable.

CARE

Testimony, advocacy, intimacy, and humanitarian aid can all contain expressions, activities, or emotions of care. The care ethos that runs throughout humanitarian action is itself a complex contradiction. Caring for unknown suffering others is central to pursuing international humanitarian aid. Such care straddles the personal and professional, as does much care work, which can be undervalued when provided by uncompensated intimates (such as parents, children, or other kin or kin-like persons), but also when provided by professionals outside of any prior intimate connection who tend to be undercompensated for their labor. The contingent "volunteer" spirit of humanitarian missions, in which expatriates are not contract employees but temporary volunteers on stipends rather than salaries, mirrors both sides of this structure of care: expatriate humanitarian workers are supposed to be mission driven, motivated by altruistic ideals and therefore undercompensated for their extreme labor, yet also to be professionals who administer care impartially, not motivated by intimate connection and affiliation, but by their role as contracted caregiver.

Ethics of care initially emerged as a response and alternate to dominant ethical theories from which women, their experiences, and the realm of the domestic sphere (home, family, motherhood) to which women were historically relegated, were excluded. Theorists like Carol Gilligan, Nel Noddings, and Eva Kittay turned to motherhood and the domestic sphere as springboard for a different kind of ethical theorizing, in which moral agents were not abstract rational agents detached from their context, but instead were situated beings, with relational obligations, and affective attachments might inform or reflect ethical reasoning, not bias or negate it. In response, other feminist theorists have challenged perceived prescriptive notions of womanhood or motherhood, worrying that certain care theories rely on and entrench women's marginalization within oppressive structures like motherhood, heteronormative relationships, caregiving, and home. For example, Tronto develops a public ethic of care that explicitly moves care theory into a political realm and political theory. The pluralism of care theory is perhaps one of its strengths, as care itself can be, as Held points out, a value, a practice, an activity, and a feeling (Held 2006).

Humanitarian care further collapses any strict assumptions about who does care work, and how. Humanitarian aid can certainly be a form of care, yet one conducted far from any sense of home, and outside classic family or kinship structures. The work is an "all-encompassing endeavor" which is not done "at home"—when carried out by expatriate workers it is nearly always done away from home, and apart from family (Fechter 2012, 1392). While certainly not true of all expatriate workers, we might also wonder how often those who build a humanitarian career in the field feel any attachment to home or a particular home in the first place. Alexander recalls hearing that "at some point many people in the aid industry continue to return to the field because they drift so far from home they no longer recognize themselves in it" (256).

In their survey of MSF retention, Korff et al. characterize aid work as involving "extreme work-family reconciliation difficulties" and initially hypothesized that women leave the humanitarian sector more frequently than men because of "parenthood and family obligations" (2015, 529) and that those in long-term relationships are less likely to re-enlist in humanitarian missions relative to those who are single due to the burdens of extended separation from partners or children (2015, 530). Yet their hypothesis regarding sex-identity did not prove true: women were no less likely to re-enlist, though relationship status at time of initial departure was significant to re-enlistment (2015, 535). Without any qualitative or reflective analysis from the surveyed cohort it is impossible to know if their initial hypothesis regarding parenthood and family obligations was untrue because such obligations were equally felt by male and female aid workers, or because male and female aid workers were equally unlikely to have such obligations in the first place, possibly making their initial enlistment in a humanitarian mission possible.

Home and away, intimacy and distance, witnessing and testimony, all join together in productive tension within care, especially when care occurs in humanitarian settings, across cultural and geographic distances. In care there is always a cared-for and a caring-one (though individuals or groups may alternately or concurrently inhabit both roles). The humanitarian project tends to construe the expatriate worker as caring-one, and the local beneficiary population or individual as the cared-for. Yet the ways in which aid work nourish and sustain (while also taxing and traumatizing) those providing it complicate any clear dichotomy between caring-one and cared-for, and the care labor local staff conduct to sustain expatriates is also a (marginalized and potentially oppressive) form of care, from cooking meals and cleaning houses to translating language and culture, and orienting and training new batches of rotating expatriates. Intimate and interpersonal relationships between expatriates and locals render the cared-for and caring-one a further porous distinction.

While it might be an obvious point, care is a relationship, whether professionalized or private, though not always, or even often a reciprocal relationship. According to Noddings, the "value I place on the relatedness of caring" is a source of moral obligation (13) governed by two criteria. One is an "absolute" condition that there is a present relationship, or the potential for one; the other is a "priority" condition informing how we prioritize our care according to the "dynamic potential" for growth of the relationship "including the potential for increased reciprocity and, perhaps, mutuality" (Noddings, 15). To understand humanitarian aid as care work situates it within a relational enterprise, drawing on the intimacy of care, while also allowing for this intimacy to be in tension, a push-pull of closeness and detachment. It also locates the special obligations of care within a relationship that ought to strive toward increased reciprocity. Reciprocity is not quid pro quo. Much like care in non-humanitarian settings, there are often disparities between needs for care and capacities to care. Medical providers in non-humanitarian settings are not expecting their patients to reciprocate by providing their medical doctor with medical care. But this does not mean there is not reciprocity or exchange in clinical encounters and care settings outside of non-humanitarian or local care contexts.

Reciprocity and mutuality are latent aims of humanitarian aid, which should strive to collaborate with and empower local communities. Yet achieving collaboration and empowerment in practice can be illusive. As Alexander's colleague said: humanitarian aid can be a take-it-or-leave-it proposition, which is far from collaborative, and one of intense power imbalance like in prison—far from reciprocal. Fechter suggests the very phenomenon of the humanitarian memoir points to the collapsing of professional and private within the lives of expatriate workers. The humanitarian memoir also centers the experience of the (usually white) worker (often from the global North). Of course, these memoirists are writing their own stories, about their personal, intellectual, and emotional growth—while everyone else, whether fellow expat, friend or family from home, or local staff or beneficiary, is a supporting player.

While care is often in some way intimate, including care toward strangers or those with whom we have not historically identified, care need not be affective or emotional. The kinds of relationships in which care occurs ideally have the potential for reciprocity and mutuality, but reciprocity and mutuality are not necessary conditions for care. Co-engagement occurs in well-modeled caring encounters, but does not hinge on affective connection, nor complete reciprocity. As noted, care often occurs in contexts where reciprocity is inhibited or impossible. I require care while I am ill, and while the care a partner provides is something I might reciprocate in the future, the care my physician provides is not. We care for our young children regardless of whether they care for us in old age (though some might hope they will).

Co-engagement, unlike strict reciprocity, suggests that all involved parties to a relationship express or acknowledge engagement, but not that they meet each other in any form of exchange, whether equal or not, mutual or not, shared or not. This might look like a situation in which an individual's expressed need for care is her engagement in a relationship in which she will not be able to reciprocate the care she requires, in which her expression of need invites another to respond through care, yielding co-engagement. Attending to the emotional registers of humanitarian care work, the complicated intimacy and testimony of, toward, and among oneself and others, creates a space for a kind of co-engagement that *could* participate in a productive de-centering of global North/white/developed nation supremacy in humanitarian action, though it can also entrench hierarchy and oppression.

The humanitarian narratives in question are told from a white, developed nation perspective, positing the white figure as the agent capable of providing aid, developing professionally and personally, and undertaking the project of internal and external reflection and critique. But recognizing how these narratives reveal layered, at times contradictory emotional and psychic registers, collapsing clear distinctions regarding intimacy, testimony, and care, affords an opportunity to further break down dichotomous attitudes toward humanitarian action itself, its methods, its self-identity, and to embrace a co-engaged posture. Co-engagement allows for the many human shortcomings we find in these memoirs, and the complexities of situated relationships (professional, personal, sexual, transactional, and caring) across difference—and distance. It supports connections among and between the diversity of experiences and emotions of others, and within the self, that occur in humanitarian caring exchanges—whether as the cared-for or caring-one, recognizing that we all will at times inhabit either or both roles, no matter our initial historical or geographical position. Care theory initially turned inward, looking to home and the domestic for insights into how care affords a unique ethical framework. Humanitarian care is by definition done elsewhere, far from home, at a distance. Yet humanitarian care shows how care done elsewhere enriches a framework for care done anywhere.

REFERENCES

Alexander, Jessica. 2013. *Chasing chaos: My decade in and out of humanitarian aid.* Broadway Books.

Bauman, Emily. 2019. "The naive republic of aid." In *Global humanitarianism and media culture*, edited by Michael Lawrence and Rachel Tavernor. Manchester University Press: 83–102.

Bowden, Peta. 1997. *Caring: Gender sensitive ethics.* London: Routledge.

Brandsen, Cheryl. 2006. "A public ethic of care: Implications for long-term care." In *Socializing care: Feminist ethics and public issues*, edited by Maurice Hamington and Dorothy C. Miller. Oxford: Rowman & Littlefield Publishers: 205–226.

Bubeck, Diemut. 1995. *Care, gender, and justice.* Oxford: Oxford University Press.

Cain, Kenneth, Heidi Postlewait and Andrew Thomson. 2004. *Emergency sex (and other desperate measures): True stories from a war zone.* Random House.

Fechter, Anne-Meike. 2012. "The personal and the professional: Aid workers' relationships and values in the development process." *Third World Quarterly* 33.8: 1387–1404.

Fyfe, Shannon and Elizabeth Lanphier. 2020. "Why ethical sex demands [the category of] nonconsensual sex." *Southwest Philosophy Review* 36.1: 135–143.

Gilligan, Carol. 1993. *In a different voice*. Cambridge, MA: Harvard University Press.
Held, Virginia. 2006. *The ethics of care*. New York: Oxford University Press, 2006.
Kittay, Eva Feder. 1999. *Love's labor: Essays on women, equality and dependency*. New York: Routledge.
Korff, Valeska P., Nicoletta Balbo, Melinda Mills, Liesbet Heyse, and Rafael Wittek. 2015. "The impact of humanitarian context conditions and individual characteristics on aid worker retention." *Disasters* 39.3: 522–545.
Lanphier, Elizabeth. 2018. "Humanitarianism: Neutrality, impartiality, and humanity." In *The Cambridge handbook of the just war,* edited by Larry May. Cambridge University Press.
Lanphier, Elizabeth. 2021. "An institutional ethic of care." In *Applying nonideal theory to bioethics: Living and dying in a nonideal world*, edited by Elizabeth Victor and Laura Guidry-Grimes. Springer.
MSF. 2020. Core ExCom message to our staff on discrimination and racism within MSF. https://www.msf.org/msf-management-statement-racism-and-discrimination
Noddings, Nel. 1984. *Caring: A feminine approach to ethics and moral education*. Berkeley: University of California Press.
Read, Róisín. 2018. "Embodying difference: Reading gender in women's memoirs of humanitarianism." *Journal of Intervention and Statebuilding* 12.3: 300–318.
Ruddick, Sara. 1998. "Care as labor and relationship." In *Norms and values: Essays on the work of Virginia Held,* edited by Mark S. Halfon and Joram C. Haber. Lanham, MD: Rowman & Littlefield.
Tronto, Joan C. 1993. *Moral boundaries*. New York: Routledge.
Tronto, Joan C. 2006. "Vicious circles of privatizing care." In *Socializing care: Feminist ethics and public issues*, edited by Maurice Hamington and Dorothy C. Miller. Oxford: Rowman & Littlefield.

Chapter 9

The Invisible Work of Care and Emotions along the Trajectories of Beninese Children Traveling to Switzerland without Their Family for Heart Surgery

Carla Vaucher

INTRODUCTION

Among the studies on medical travel (Roberts & Scheper-Hugues, 2011; Marsters, 2012; Bochaton, 2010; Lunt et al., 2015), very few of them concern the medical mobilities of children (Sakoyan, 2010; Vindrola-Padros, 2011; Massimo et al., 2008), and even fewer relate to the movement of children residing in countries of the Global South (Johnson & Vindrola-Padros, 2014). As noted by Vindrola-Padros & Bages (2016), the relevant literature is even more sparse when it comes to documenting how the children themselves experience their own medical travel, with most studies accounting for the experience of family members or health professionals.

Furthermore, while a part of the medical travel literature focuses on the liberal choices of Western people to travel abroad in order to get cheaper, higher quality, or even more restful treatment for their disease or that of a relative, Roberts and Scheper Hugues (2011:2) remind us that many people who travel for medical reasons come from economically disadvantaged backgrounds, and are "desperately seeking life-saving drugs and therapies and corrective surgeries that they cannot get at home," as is the case with the patients my research concerns. As such, the work of Kangas (2007:295) also highlights the fact that "technological medicine is more than a consumer good. Wrapped up with life and death, it is an emotional and moral good as well." Studying medical travel thus also means considering the health inequalities that exist between the different medical travelers around the world (Faist, 2013).

Finally, while the scarce literature on children's medical travel attests to the fact that children are generally accompanied by at least one family member during the course of their travels (Vindrola-Padros & Bages, 2016; Massimo et al., 2008), in the context of my research, children aged 0 to 18 travel alone, without any relatives. I have not yet found any other study that focuses on the medical travel of children without family members.

At a time when the presence of significant others–especially parents–is valued in the field of pediatrics (Lombart, 2015; Massimo et al., 2008; Mougel, 2013, 2007) and considering that the detrimental influence of a prolonged separation between children and their parents–especially in situations of illness and hospitalization–has been shown (Bowlby, 1980; Spitz, 1945), caring for these children creates unprecedented situations, practically as well as emotionally. Indeed, medical travels affect not only the young patients/travelers themselves, but also their kin, their friends, the health authorities in both countries (Vindrola-Padros & Johnson, 2015; Kangas, 2010), NGO workers, health professionals, volunteers, or other children they meet in health facilities. In this chapter, I would like to explore how the care and treatment of these children thus constitute the heart of a complex network of emotions and care work for all the actors who support them at all stages of their biographical and therapeutic trajectories.

While the literature on medical travel has mainly focused on the reasons for travel, the flow of patients around the world, or certain difficulties caused by such travel (Sobo 2009 in Johnson & Vindrola-Padros 2014), this chapter will examine the emotions experienced by the constellation of actors who plot the course of Beninese children's medical travels to Switzerland, and the work of care that both arises from these emotions and sometimes causes them, depending on the situation. The nature as well as the temporality of these emotions differ according to the individuals concerned.

The purpose of this chapter is to highlight that, in parallel with the cultural, political, medical, institutional, or even economic challenges that fall to the humanitarian specialized care program in question, and underlying the gigantic coordination work which makes it run, the emotions and care work of the different actors in a child's medical trajectory form another layer which is less often investigated and less recognized. While the surgeons' work is generally in the spotlight (without wanting to devalue it), I suggest that the emotions and care work of all the actors involved in the medical travel of children, which go beyond protocols and are not necessarily seen, recognized, or discussed by the work teams, also constitute a driving force of the program and should be made more visible.

Among the actors who participate in the medical trajectory of the children accounted for in this chapter, I would like to emphasize that the children themselves provide considerable (care) work as part of their own journey in care. By considering children as social actors (Christensen & Prout, 2002), and accounting for their emotions, care work, practices, and perceptions, I wish to contribute to acknowledging that "they, too, tailor global health, humanitarian, and biomedical systems of knowledge and practice to their particular circumstances" (Hunleth, 2017:4).

RESEARCH BACKGROUND

My doctoral thesis in the field of medical anthropology, from which this chapter stems, is devoted to the experience of Beninese children suffering from congenital heart defects, as part of their care by a humanitarian specialized care program in Switzerland. The program has existed for sixty years, has changed little since its creation, and has never been subject to an in-depth study. This program consists of welcoming children from so-called disadvantaged families from a dozen countries in West and North Africa, for surgical operations in University hospitals in Switzerland (and in rarer cases, in France and Spain). The program was created in response to a health context in which the treatment of these defects is limited by the impossibility of access to a surgical operation, due to the lack of local technical resources. It is thus thanks to non-governmental medical humanitarian aid organizations that the therapeutic projects of these children can be undertaken (Brousse et al., 2007), knowing that each medical transfer abroad generate very high costs. Beside this, while pediatric heart patients receive timely intervention in Western countries, children suffering from heart defects in West Africa are "diagnosed very late due to limited paediatric medicine infrastructure and a lack of specialised medical centres," also delaying their surgical intervention (Heinisch et al., 2019).

Upstream work is carried out by the collaborators of local delegations with the aim of evaluating the economic and social situations of families applying for the program. Once the application has been accepted, all the children's medical travel is covered by the NGO and by partner associations. Therefore, the families do not contribute financially to travel, accommodation, food, medical, or surgical costs. However, they spend significant sums of money, given their economic situations, during the medical and administrative procedures surrounding the application.

Children up to eighteen travel alone, without any family member. They are accompanied by different volunteers during their flights and movements while in Switzerland, and live in a residential care facility for children, along with about forty others, during their approximately two- to three-month stay.

Within this program, I was interested in the ways in which these children experience their illness, their heart operation, and their travel to Switzerland; how they communicated and cohabited with the various actors who crossed their path as part of their medical and social care, including other children; and how they developed communication strategies and adaptive behaviors in environments which, for several reasons, are not familiar to them.

My fieldwork within the NGO specialized care program took place between July 2018 and March 2020. My approach included participant observation as well as semi-structured interviews with children, their parents, NGO workers, and volunteers, at all stages and in all the places traveled by the children as part of their therapeutic itinerary in Benin, in Switzerland, and in-between during the flights, as well as the analysis of internal documentation and written correspondence between different agents of the program. In view of the fact that I was subjected to multiple movements in the same way as the children whose trajectories I studied, and that I made observations including during their mobilities, I consider this special kind of multi-site ethnography as an *itinerant ethnography* (see Laurier et al., 2008). The data were subject to inductive thematic analysis, making it possible to highlight both longitudinal and transverse axes concerning the children's trajectories. Pseudonyms are used for all persons quoted in this chapter.

By the end of the data collection phase, I collaborated more closely with the NGO officials, in order to discuss ways of translating my research findings into changes in practice and policy, sharing the opinion that social sciences can contribute to improving the conditions of research subjects, in this case children and their families (Vindrola Padros, Pfister & Johnson, 2015), but also volunteers and NGO and health professionals. The modalities we have discussed include a summary of my observations punctuated by suggestions for improvement, discussion groups and training for volunteers, and thematic workshops for reflection on the professionals' practices, depending on the needs and interests of each work team.

FROM THE FIRST SYMPTOMS TO THE ANNOUNCEMENT OF THE DIAGNOSIS

Although each history of a child's disease and medical travel are experienced in singular ways by the children and their families (Vindrola-Padros & Bages, 2016), for the majority of the families I met during my fieldwork in Benin, the NGO specialized care program seemed to represent a last resort option after having already been through a long and trying care journey. These trajectories were generally punctuated with numerous appointments with different physicians in several medical centers, progressive referral to cardiologists, and then orientation to the NGO program, which only meant the beginning of another journey that would also include its share of formalities, time, and concerns.

The announcement of the diagnosis of congenital heart defect was always a very emotional moment for parents and other close kin. The shock caused by the announcement of a disease requiring intricate surgery was coupled with the announcement that it would require treatment abroad as part of the NGO program, and finally that the medical travel would require separation between the child and their family for a few months. Ruben's mother recounts the shock she experienced when her child, who was only a few months old at the time, was diagnosed with a heart disease:

> I did not understand anything. My child was in my arms, and I was so disoriented I almost dropped him. The doctor repeated to me: "with what your child has, he has to have surgery. He must be operated on to stay alive." I learned that my baby had a hole in his heart, and that he needed to have an operation, in order that he would live!!! There are no words to describe how I felt, I was wrecked. There are really no words. I wouldn't even wish it on my enemy.

These different announcements and the mixed emotions they caused sometimes delayed the administrative procedure of asking for help from the NGO, as the parents often needed time to make the decision. Doubts assailed them during the procedures leading to the child's departure, as the mother of Lilly, eight months old at the time, testified: "It was super stressful and I even thought about whether to do it or not, if it was worth it." It is by putting aside her own emotions that this mother managed to make the decision to allow the medical travel of her daughter, as she explained, one week before Lilly's departure: "We must do this for her. We must think of her, of her own growth. That is why it is worth it to keep going with the procedures."

Since the diagnosis of congenital heart defect was not very well-known in the general population in Benin, a feeling of guilt was common among parents, especially among mothers, who wondered and were often judged as to the origin of their child's disease. During the same interview, one week before Lilly's departure, both her parents shared with me their doubts and questions about this. While this couple reassured themselves by telling themselves that they had undergone all the recommended medical examinations and dietary restrictions during the mother's pregnancy, Ruben's mother testified in more detail to her feeling of guilt, produced by the accusations of those around her, including her husband:

I asked the cardiologist what caused the disease; was it because of my diet during pregnancy? Had I made a mistake, had I taken a medication that I shouldn't have? What happened? He reassured me and told me it had nothing to do with my diet, that it was a natural phenomenon. I also thought that maybe it was a divine punishment. I asked myself, why me? Does heaven blame me for something? You know, in Africa, it's hard to explain to people that your first born has a disease. My mother-in-law told me: "Look inside yourself and ask yourself, my daughter, whether it is possible that before meeting my son, you did stupid things . . . And if this is the case, it is normal that your child has this problem." And with many people, even if it is not in their words, you feel in their behaviour that they blame you for something. At first, you know, I'm not going to lie to you, when we got married, my husband didn't want a child right away. After some negotiations, he got me pregnant. So, when the child was born, like that, sick, it was a shock for him. At first, he didn't want a child, I practically forced him, and then the child came, but sick. Immediately he started to accuse me: "You see, it's because you were in a hurry. We did not wait for the right time. You weren't patient. It wasn't God's time, but you insisted." He made me feel guilty for a while.

Although the cardiologists explicitly told the parents that they had no responsibility for their child's disease and that congenital heart defects happened by accident everywhere in the world, it did not prevent the fathers as well as those around the family from making the mother feel guilty afterwards, or even during the same appointment in the presence of the cardiologist.

Despite the great concerns generated by their child's disease and by their future medical travel, parents mostly felt lucky to be offered the opportunity to heal their child, as Ruben's mother explained: "The fact that my child would heal gave me the strength to complete all the formalities for him to travel. Since this opportunity existed, I told myself that I would not miss it. For nothing in the world should I miss it. Other mothers would have liked to have had this opportunity for their children. If I had this opportunity and did not take it, I would be ungrateful to my God." As Sobo (2015:224) suggests and as the above quotation seems to highlight, "undertaking medical travel can serve as a demonstration of social position [. . .] [and as a way to] create and maintain [one's] identities as 'good' relatives."

Many concerns arose as the child's departure date approached, in particular relating to the length of their stay in Europe, and the way in which parents and children would experience separation, as Lilly's parents explained:

Father: On the one hand, there is uncertainty, we do not know. Because they [NGO employees] say it is often three months. But the operation can last, and it can go beyond six months, even one year. Up to a year, well I wonder if your child, who left while she was a baby, will recognize you. Nothing is easy, everything is complicated, anyway.

Mother: Absence will always be absence. We will try to endure it in our own way. Because for me, well, she is my hobby. I do practically nothing at all, we are together all the time. So, I will try to kill time, look for something to do so as not to feel her absence too much.

SUPPORT AND SOLIDARITY NETWORKS

Benin is one of the rare member countries of the program where an association has been created, on the initiative of the local employees of the NGO and of parents whose children have traveled previously, in order to support families in the process of separation during the child's medical travel. As such, on each departure and each return to Benin, families whose children had benefited from the program in the past and ex-officio members of the association were present at the airport and supported the families of the children who were about to leave or return. Support was expressed by families sharing their stories, memories, or photographs of their children, before and after their medical travel, and by distracting parents with anecdotes, or by comforting them. Ruben's mother shared what the association changed for her, as she was preparing for her son's departure, in these words:

> Knowing that, from now on, you have people who have had the same experience as you, who have cried as you have, for the same cause, who have fought, who have hoped, finally who have triumphed, people who practically shared your story, who have lived the same things as you, you tell yourself: they are my family. Because you have a lot to tell each other. It is a family, from now on. And each time I see them, I am happy, I feel at home.

A GENDERED FACET OF EMOTIONS

During my observations of the preparations related to the departure of a child, I noted that the interpretation of emotions as well as their management by the people around the parents were gendered in structure. Indeed, more attention as well as more support seemed to be given to the mother of the child, rather than to the father, an attitude relying on the perception that the mothers' emotions were more legitimate that those of the father. When the parents of two-year-old Joshua came to the NGO office, on the same day Joshua would leave for Switzerland, the father told the NGO employee that he had no appetite since he knew his child had to leave for medical reasons.

The employee answered: "You have to imagine what the mother is going to go through, because the child stayed with her all the time." Despite the fact that the father's emotions were not legitimized in this conversation with the employee, the latter however took them into account at the end of the interview, when he said: "I do not want to take the risk of having you drive in this state, so we will drive you to the airport tonight." As such, I had the impression that attention to the fathers' emotions was reflected more in actions to protect them from reckless acts, while attention to mothers' emotions was expressed with empathetic questions, and physical or verbal reassurance.

The perception that the separation was more difficult for the mother than for the father was shared by the members of the association who accompanied six-year-old Maya's family on the evening of her departure. A father whose child had traveled to Europe previously explained to me that the members of the association were also here to "distract the parents, to bring a little joy in this difficult moment." He added: "Above all, you have to talk with the mother a lot. Because she is the one who carried and fed the child, and even if it looks like she is listening, in reality she is absent, she is thinking about her child, and she will shed tears once she is home. Even now she is in the car, shedding tears."

During my fieldwork at the airport, I noticed that the fathers' emotions, while more discreet, were still observable. In most situations, the emotions of both parents were contained and rather discreet in the public area which is the airport. Social conventions seemed to prevail over the expression of negative emotions, as in the case of Maya's departure when her parents continued to talk and smile when spoken to, although staring blankly.

BEHIND THE SCENES OF EMOTIONS

While the emotions of the children and the families are obvious and recognized as legitimate, despite their efforts to hide them in public most of the time, the emotions of other actors are considered less so, and require constant emotional labor (Hochschild, 1983). This is the case for the NGO employees in Benin as well as in Switzerland, but also for the volunteers, for the health professionals in both countries, and for me, as a researcher.

Managing One's Own Emotions as Well as the Emotions of Others

The professionals who worked for the NGO in Benin supported the families on a daily and long-term basis. They accompanied them in their administrative procedures, during medical appointments, and supported them morally through their trajectory. They personally knew the parents, the child in need of medical care and their siblings, sometimes the grandparents or other members of the family, and they developed friendly and sometimes almost familial ties. They kept in touch before, during and after the child's medical travel.

The occasions when the emotions of professionals appeared to me most clearly were the days of children's departures, which generally occurred once or twice per week. To avoid emotional exhaustion, the professionals in Benin had deliberately decided to take turns.

> On the day of Lilly's departure, after NGO employee Sarah has taken care of relaying Lilly to the volunteer who will accompany her during her flight, she comes back to the family and says that "everything went well" and that she will call them the next morning to inform them of Lilly's arrival in Switzerland. We say goodbye to the family and leave. Directly after, on the way to the carpark, Sarah tells me it was a really tough departure. She says that the baby girl cried a lot, that they passed her from arm to arm, that she was disoriented. Once in the car, Sarah sits at the front, leans forward, puts her hand on her forehead, and sniffs. I put my hand on her shoulder and ask her if she is okay. She takes a moment to answer and says: "I'm fine." When she turns around, I see that she has tears in her eyes. Then she adds: "you must be able to hold out in front of the family." The 10-minute drive then takes place in total silence.

This excerpt shows that the professionals had to deal with their own emotions as well as with the emotions of others, and that they repressed the expression of their own emotions in front of the families. But this emotional labor had consequences, as the professionals took their emotions home with them. One week after Lilly's departure, as Sarah was about to coordinate another departure, we left the office together. In the street in front of the building, she told me: "I hope that tonight's separation will go well. Last week, it really wasn't easy for me. I didn't sleep all night because I was imagining how things were going for Lilly."

Furthermore, the professionals' emotions did not arise only at children's departures, when they had to manage the separation between a child and their parents. Their emotional involvement was constant. One professional, James, summed it up: "We are not only dealing with files, they are not papers. We are dealing with humans." James told me about the difficulty of their daily work, and said it's emotionally exhausting, and that sometimes he wonders if he should quit. He told me about situations where families come to the office and their child's case does not meet the NGO criteria and where he has to refuse their application, and about the mother kneeling in front of him and imploring him. He said that in front of families he holds out, but that sometimes in the evening he can no longer hold it all back.

Just a few days later, when I arrived at the office in the morning, another employee, Raphael, informed me that he had just received a call from parents to inform them that their child had died, while his medical transfer to Switzerland was scheduled soon after. He then told me: "Now there is no one to comfort us." Many cases showed that taking care of families' emotions weighed on the NGO professionals, who would have benefited from emotional support, too. In Switzerland also, the NGO employees' emotional burden was high, although in a different way, as they were not confronted with the children's families. However, NGO workers went to greet the children at the airport on the day of their arrival and drove them to the hospitals. While I accompanied Sandra one day as she was driving a child to the hospital, she confessed to me: "You have to be strong. You get used to it as you go. But there are still situations that affect me. Recently, I collapsed when I learnt about the death of a child." As I followed her work, I saw signs of her progressive exhaustion. Although not seeing the children very much, the NGO workers knew all the details of their medical trajectory and got attached to them, sometimes visiting them at the hospital although their professional function did not require them to do so.

Experiencing the Limits of Their Function

Both in Benin and in Switzerland, health professionals experienced the limits of their function when they were confronted with difficulties in caring for the children within the humanitarian medicine program. In Benin, the shortcomings of the health system were felt above all in relation to the lack of necessary equipment as well as skilled personnel for the treatment of congenital heart defects. To make up for the lack of on-site training, doctors who wanted to specialize in pediatric cardiology were often trained in Europe, as is the case with a cardiologist who told me about his frustration with local resources: "We encounter many difficulties related to the imprecision of diagnoses, due to the lack of specialized training and adequate equipment." But limits were also felt due to the contrast between the willingness of the cardiologists and the slow administrative pace of the NGO: according to the same cardiologist, "one problem is the delay between the submission of an application and the child's medical travel. Sometimes the children die in the meantime. It is a huge burden for us."

In Switzerland, the emotions of health professionals stem more from the fact that hospital partnerships with humanitarian programs require them to take care of children who do not necessarily speak the same language as them, and who are not accompanied by their parents. Massimo et al. (2008) have reported similar difficulties in verbal communication in the context of caring for foreign children in an Italian pediatric oncology service. During my observations in hospital settings, the nursing staff kept asking me if I had information on the eating or sleeping habits of these children or on the way babies were usually carried, revealing both their perception of a shift in cultural practices, and the absence of a link in the care chain. An intensive care unit manager shared her thoughts with me: "The biggest problem with these children is the fact that we lack an intermediary representing the child, a link between the child and us, namely the parents, as we have for the other children we welcome in the unit." The caregivers also told me that they felt empathy, even pity, for these children who were hospitalized without their parents. To compensate for the perceived lack, the caregivers adopted parental postures, filled with tenderness toward these children. For example, as she prepared to undergo a cardiac catheterization exam, three-year-old Clementine was carried in an anesthesiologist's arms. A nurse passed by and kissed her on the cheek. Clementine snuggled against the anesthesiologist's shoulder. This observation shows that both caregivers and children adapted to the absence of parents: caregivers by adopting a more parental posture, and children by seeking physical contact with caregivers.

Despite the fact that the caregivers appreciated the mutual tenderness with the children, they mostly felt helpless and had feelings of guilt over the fact that they could not be around the children all the time, despite the children's needs. This was especially the case for nurses. Nurses also developed protective and advocating attitudes toward the children and granted them small privileges, more so than was the case with children accompanied by their parents during their hospital stay. On one of my first days of observation in the baby unit, I asked two nurses if the children cared for by the NGO were considered the same as the other regular patients. They immediately reacted very strongly, saying that these children "had many more rights than the others," and that the nurses "had a much more parental attitude towards them": "we are their advocates, too." They said that they took them with them during their lunch breaks and in the nurses' office, defended them against the doctors, for example, by asking if it was really necessary to have them do blood tests every day, and that they were also more forgiving with them.

The Thankless Care Work of Volunteers

When traveling by plane to and from Switzerland, the children were accompanied by volunteers from a different NGO. Due to the lack of time and the administrative procedures to be completed, volunteers generally met the children they would accompany only about 15 minutes before going through the security gates with them. Sometimes they did not even meet their family before leaving with the children. When leaving in stress due to a flight delay, one volunteer confessed to me: "I would have liked to meet the family before. When it happens like this, I feel like a child kidnapper."

Time and organizational constraints had a direct effect both on the volunteers and the children's experience, and thus on the way the journey unfolded. For the children, as they sometimes did not have time to get used to the person who would accompany them, the beginning of the journey sometimes took place in panic and tears, which put volunteers in uncomfortable positions, especially with regards to other passengers on the flight. This discomfort was compounded by the fact that other passengers were not aware of the exact situation, and allowed themselves questions, comments, and judgments. On his arrival at Geneva airport when entrusting 18-month-old Imany and nine-year-old Laura to the NGO employee, a tired volunteer confided: "On the plane, it was difficult; at the beginning, Imany cried a lot. Everyone was looking at me, and people asked the flight attendants why I was the one taking care of these children, and why it wasn't a woman who was traveling with them. People thought I was stealing children." Once again, this shows the gendered perceptions attached to care work, as well as the feelings of the lack of legitimacy of the volunteer work.

The journeys in Switzerland, for example between the children's place of accommodation and the hospitals, were also dealt with by volunteers. Although they spent limited time together, volunteers and children nevertheless developed a certain attachment, which made separation sometimes difficult for both parties. In the long run, volunteers, like professionals working for the NGO, learned to "armour themselves," as they put it.

Unraveling the Researcher's Emotions

Several authors have addressed the fact that the researchers' emotions are not sufficiently considered in the analysis of the research process, and that they do not testify enough to the part played by emotional dimensions in the production of knowledge (Brannan, 2011; Pirinoli, 2004). In a recent article (Vaucher, 2020a), I reflected on how the researcher's reflexivity regarding his or her own emotions during fieldwork could contribute to an approach that is both epistemological and ethical. In this previous article, I focused mainly on the emotions related to my research posture, namely a kind of dissonance between my "researcher identity" and my "personal identity," at the same time questioning the fact that there are two clearly distinct identities.

Here, I wish to focus more on the emotions I experienced in contact with the children during the days spent with them, and in particular in the context of observing the care and examinations they underwent in a hospital setting. My emotions were closely linked to the very committed posture

I adopted during my fieldwork, as most of the time, I occupied the role of a reference person, or even a parental substitute for the children. Very quickly at the beginning of my fieldwork, I noticed that I experienced a kind of emotional empathy toward the children whom I accompanied, as I frequently had tears in my eyes when watching a child cry during a blood test or a vaccine. I interpreted my reaction as a response to the fact that I was aware of the entire social and medical trajectory of these children, and was, therefore, able to imagine the depth of their emotions, which I perceived as going beyond the mere moment of the blood test or injection. Gallenga (2008:4) suggests that the notion of empathy should be inscribed at the heart of the definition of anthropology, or considered as an ethnographic method, as one of the main aims of anthropology is to produce knowledge about others.

I mostly experienced sadness as well as helplessness when I visited young children in the baby unit, and found them sitting in their crib, watching for any movement in the hallway. Several times, when I took them in my arms, they immediately snuggled against my neck, searching for skin-to-skin contact, and quickly fell asleep to the sound of my lullabies. I also felt terribly sad when I tried to play with a child who was apathetic due to medication, or suspicious because they mistook me for a member of the healthcare team. Feelings of guilt very often inhabited me, surfacing almost each time I had to leave the hospital at the end of the day and leave a child alone. As my fieldwork progressed and I could no longer bare the imploring gazes of children when I left their room, I got into the habit of leaving during their naps. This strategy spared me painful separations, but not the feelings of guilt. Indeed, on the train back home, I wondered what the children would think when they woke up, whether they would feel betrayed or that I had abandoned them.

Despite my great emotional fatigue after the days I spent in hospitals, I noticed that the emotions I experienced guided me in the field, leading me to occupy roles and functions that I would not have occupied without them. Thanks to this fully committed position, I had access to unexpected situations which offered me additional insight into my research object. One day when I had only planned to observe the arrival of two-year old Kenzo at the airport, the tenderness and the joy I experienced in the presence of this boy, who had an apoplexy crisis and who had to be transported by ambulance to the hospital, but who was still playing with a teddy bear and laughing in the ambulance when his life was threatened, as well as the fear I felt for his medical condition, led me to accompany him to the emergency room, to spend the whole morning with him, and finally to access the operating room where I was able to attend his entire heart operation. This was the one and only time I was admitted in the operating room.

Finally, despite the fact that positive emotions seemed more difficult to circumscribe in my fieldnotes, I must nonetheless do them justice, as I have experienced many of these as well. The next excerpt shows one of these situations:

> I visited two-year old Nayel at the intensive care unit, three days after his operation, and I found him motionless and listless in his bed, his eyes open just a crack. At the same time, a volunteer musician entered the room, and came to play kalimba music at his bedside. Nayel began to move his fingers gently while looking carefully at the musician, as if he were playing the same instrument himself. While continuing to move his fingers to the sound of the music, he started to move his legs under the blanket, struggling to keep his eyes open. His nurse approached and the three of us stood at his bedside, smiling at this moving scene, in a soft and benevolent atmosphere.

CHILDREN'S EMOTIONS BEFORE THEIR MEDICAL TRAVEL

In general, children were surprisingly absent in the process surrounding the preparation of their travels. Indeed, although they were systematically present during the medical and administrative procedures, little or no room was given for the expression of their thoughts or emotions. This was partly due to local perceptions in West Africa that the child does not have the right to speak unless asked to, as well as to the idea that the child should not be involved in "negative" situations, as the NGO professionals and some parents explained to me. Previous research has shown that in West African cultures, children mostly have to ask permission to speak in the presence of adults, a posture described by Jaffré et al. (2009:244) as the child being ""the s/he" of an interaction; the one people are talking about, but to whom no one is talking." [author's translation]. As a result, the face-to-face interviews I conducted with several children represented rare opportunities for the children to speak about their personal experience in relation to their disease and their medical travel.

One week before her departure, Victoria, 16 years old, told me: "I am happy to go there, to be healed and come back home safe and sound. I hope that the doctors there will be nice." Although Victoria's speech was full of hope regarding her recovery, the fear of separation from her family, especially her mother, quickly became apparent: "When my mom doesn't see me, she is sad. For me, it is the same: when I don't see my mom, I am sad. I pray God will give me the confidence to stay alone and not worry about my mom so much. And I pray for her that my older brother's wife can come and stay with her for a while."

Surprisingly, fear about separation outweighed fears about her disease or her future heart surgery. This excerpt also shows the gendered aspect of domestic work and recalls that when a child leaves the country for some time, the separation is not only difficult for the parents emotionally, but it can also be difficult in practice, since children, even when sick, provide daily domestic work. The work of Hunleth in Zambia (2017:136) has shown how children can also assume household and nurturing work when their relatives are sick, and that a gendered sense of responsibility can be observed at a young age.

During interviews, sometimes conducted retrospectively after the child's return, some children expressed their joy of traveling to Europe, sometimes equating their medical travel with a touristic trip, such as Antonio, 14 years old, who I met in Benin almost one month after his return from France: "I was happy to leave because I had never seen France before. I had heard of it, and of the Eiffel Tower. So, I went to France for my operation . . . and some memories."

CARING FOR EACH OTHER DURING THEIR MEDICAL TRAVEL: CHILDREN'S EMOTIONAL AND CARE WORK

As shown above, the start of the children's journey was often tormented. While the youngest were frequently anxious and cried a lot, the older ones mostly hid in silence. When children recounted their experiences to me, they often remembered their fear of flying, as 14-year-old Agatha remembered: "When I had to get on the plane, I was afraid." This fear, while expected in children who have never taken a plane before, also arose in other less obvious situations, like, for example, when the children were afraid to get in an elevator or to take an escalator in the airports and held on to my arm nervously.

In another publication (Vaucher, 2020b), I described the care practices that the children deployed among themselves during their stay in Switzerland within their residential care facility. The care interactions between children of different ages and different nationalities included forms of socialization with the rules of the hosting facility and life in the community in general, practical help, aesthetic care and hygiene, moral support, tenderness, solidarity, translating and mediating the words and moods of other children, or expressing interest and concern for other children, and their medical trajectory. The article sheds a light on a model of socialization and care between children and shows that children can be both recipients and providers of care. This observation is similar to that of Vindrola-Padros & Johnson (2015:1) who underlined that children could be both "independent agents looking after their own health and well-being and family dependents with competing responsibilities [. . .] [such as providing for] younger siblings." In the context of my study, the children's competing responsibilities complexified as they could relate both to their family of origin and to the "strong sense of kinship" they developed toward their "temporary surrogate family" (Ackerman, 2010:418) constituted by other children experiencing similar life situations in Switzerland.

I have observed that these forms of care could also be found at other stages of the children's trajectories, for instance, during flights or at the hospital:

> At 16-year-old Victoria and two-year-old Safira's departure, more than an hour after the plane took off, Safira is still struggling and yelling stridently. I show her magazines, try to sing her a song, rock her, nothing helps. She screams and struggles for no apparent reason. Victoria looks at me helplessly and says to me: "She is afraid." After a while, Safira puts two fingers in her mouth and falls asleep for a moment but is quickly disturbed by a flight attendant who brings the meal trays and she starts to cry again. Victoria takes her in her arms, and places Safira's fingers back in her mouth the same way she saw her do it earlier. Safira goes back to sleep. Victoria keeps her on her lap for a moment and then manages to put her in her seat without waking her.

This excerpt shows both mediation care work, tainted with a probable projection of her own feelings when Victoria interprets Safira's cries as fear, and practical help and solicitude to soothe Safira. Similar care work between children was observed at the hospital, as shown in the two following excerpts:

> 10-year-old Laura and 18-month-old Imany are undergoing an initial health check-up at the hospital on the day of their arrival in Switzerland. As a doctor tries to take Imany's temperature, she screams and struggles, pushing away the doctor's arm. Laura, who was sitting on her own bed, gets up, approaches her and tries to comfort her by tapping on her stomach gently.

Despite the fact that care from girls, and from older children toward younger ones was more frequent, I also observed situations of care from boys, and from younger children toward older ones, as in this scene:

> On the day of nine-year-old Theo and two-year-old William's arrival in Switzerland, and while undergoing their initial check-up, William walks happily through the hospital corridors, plays and laughs with the caregivers, while Theo looks serious, remaining motionless and mute. We go to the dining room, where William starts to eat with appetite and pleasure. Theo barely tastes his plate, head down. William looks at him and says: "Eat! Come on, eat!" Theo sobs while eating a few pieces of pasta, drinks a very small sip of water, and then leaves his entire meal tray.

The care practices deployed between children also extended to care toward adults, and in particular their families, despite the distance.

> When he has been in Switzerland for two months, 10-year-old Jacob is sitting at his desk in the classroom, and when I sit next to him, he spontaneously tells me: "I am worried about my mom, that she has problems with her work, because she is alone taking care of us. My father does not work."

As other authors have shown before, children experiencing illness and/or medical travel perceive the economic, emotional, and social burdens they place on their families and the consequences this can generate, sometimes leading to feelings of guilt (Vindrola-Padros & Whiteford, 2012; Vindrola-Padros & Brage, 2016; Couturier, 2019).

CHILDREN'S MIXED FEELINGS

The first days after the arrival of a child in Switzerland were often difficult, with children having to get used to new places, new faces, sometimes to new languages, and practices. Sobbing attacks and difficulty falling asleep were thus frequent in the children's residential care facility. Mixed emotions animated the children, between the joy of discovering that they were not alone in their situation, the sadness of missing their families, and the fear of going to the hospital and seeing the date of their operation approaching. During an interview with ten-year-old Maria, three days after her return to Benin, she recalled her fear of undergoing heart surgery and how the educational staff reassured her: "When I was at the house [residential care facility], they [educational staff] said that they [at the hospital] were going to operate on me. I was afraid. And the people who work at the house they told me not to be afraid, that it would not be complicated, they said don't be so sad."

Memories related to the operation itself were rare in children's speech. However, they frequently spoke of their surprise or fear when they discovered their chest scar, as well as the boredom and sadness of being alone at the hospital. It was sometimes also difficult for the children to understand why the other children hospitalized in the same service were visited by their parents when they were not. The following excerpt of my hospital fieldwork shows this confusion:

> As six-year-old Mila and I move from the service playroom to her room, we meet a group of people in the corridor: a child, his parents, and a nurse. Apparently, the child is about to leave the hospital. The father takes him in his arms, and the

child seems very happy. I try to motivate Mila to move towards her room, but she remains frozen, next to me, leaning against the wall, and seems to want to observe the scene. When everyone leaves, she asks me, with the little French she masters: "Why mom and dad? Me also mom and dad leave?" I explain to her that unfortunately not, that she will see them when she flies back home. As I have to leave, I then accompany her to the nurses' office. She sits on a nurse's laps and snuggles against her chest.

Over the time spent in the residential care facility, the children developed friendships with other children, as well as attachments to the educational, nursing, cooking, and cleaning staff. Therefore, when the time came to leave the hosting facility in order to return to their country of origin, farewells could sometimes be as painful as arrivals.

THE RETURN OF THE CHILD: FROM JOY TO DIFFICULTY

When the children returned to Benin, the first emotions experienced by parents and other family members were joy, followed by surprise in relation to physical and capacity changes noticed in the children. During an interview, Ruben's mother remembered the day of his return to Benin:

> I asked permission to quickly come home from work. When I got home, I prepared everything, I cleaned everywhere, I went shopping and bought him a lot of clothes, and I made him garlands, everywhere I wrote "welcome back, my child," "mom loves you," "I'm happy," "Now I am a mother," as if he could read! [. . .] When I saw him at the airport, he was chubby and beautiful! I said: "Ruben, is that you?" He didn't even look at me! I said: "It is mom, I am here." I wanted to take him in my arms, first he didn't want to, and then—you know here in Benin we have litanies, everyone has a litany here, so I reminded him of it, and at that moment he opened his arms to me. I was very happy.

As in this excerpt, it was frequent that the children did not jump into their parents' arms immediately upon arrival, as could be expected, and were a little wary at first, especially when they were babies or young children. Returns were sometimes not as happy as one would imagine due to the relationships the children had developed in Switzerland, and the difficulty of this new separation for them, as was the case for 10-year-old Maria, who arrived in tears at Cotonou airport, when she met with her mother and brother, and said she was sad to have left a friend in Switzerland, and that she would have liked for her to have come back on the same flight.

After a few days, children sometimes found it hard to get used to local rhythms and customs, reminding us that "medical travel is an inherently cross-cultural exercise" (Sobo, 2015:225).

> Four days after six-year-old Marc-Antoine's return to Benin, he and his mother come to the NGO office for a return interview. While I knew Marc-Antoine as a rather talkative and joyful boy in Switzerland and during the journey back to Benin, I immediately notice that he is discreet and silent at the office. While his mother speaks with the social worker, James, Marc-Antoine sits motionless, his head lowered to the ground. The social worker asks the mother: "How have you found him this weekend?" She answers "fine" but looks pretty desperate. James enquires: "Did something go wrong?" She answers: "He won't eat. Nothing." James reassures her: "It takes a little time to get used to our meals." The mother also says that Marc-Antoine asked her why people in the neighbourhood were staring at him, and that she told him it was because he had changed. The mother concludes: "It is not easy."

As we can see, for the parents and family members, the pain due to the child's absence, and the joy of having their child back, was sometimes quickly replaced by distress or annoyance when they realized that their child had changed, sometimes in relation to educational models that contradicted their own. Six months after 16-year-old Victoria's return to Benin, her mother told me about her perception of the changes in her daughter since her return: "She has changed completely! In all ways. Ah! She has completely changed. Really, even when she speaks now, she speaks without thinking, just like that. Where is the respect, really? This is why I get angry often. I ask: 'what is going on? Since you came back, what's wrong? There is no more respect, what is that, what is happening?!'" Three days after 10-year-old Maria's return to Benin, her mother also told me how her daughter had developed new habits since she returned from Switzerland: "She got used to brushing her teeth after breakfast. When she wakes up in the morning, I say: 'Maria, come and brush your teeth' and she answers: 'No mother, I have to eat first. When I finish eating, then I will go brush my teeth'." Victoria's and Maria's behaviors both challenged their mothers' authority. Furthermore, they show a circulation of educative and hygiene standards.

During the interviews after their return, children told me how happy they were to be healthy and to be able to do things that they could not do before because of their disease, as thirteen-year-old Constance explained, twenty-five days after her return: "Before, I couldn't walk, I was lying down all the time. Now I'm walking well. Just before coming here today, my mom asked me to go buy some supplies, and I am very happy about that. It's like I've been born again. Because everything I could not do, now I can do it."

Constance's speech shows that her joy also came from her rediscovered social role, as a young girl capable of helping her parents with domestic tasks, which once again highlights the part played by children in care work. However, although they said they were happy to be back with their families and to see their classmates again, some children also expressed a will to return to Switzerland. Six months after her return, a little embarrassed, Victoria told me: "Since I have returned, it has been good. But sometimes I also want to go back there. I miss the friends I had there and the other people, too. And sometimes the food, also." The desire to return was also present in younger children, as in the case of six-year-old Marc-Antoine. One week after his return to Benin, during a follow-up appointment with a cardiologist, Marc-Antoine's mother told the doctor: "He says he wants to go back already." During my interview with Marc-Antoine a few days later, as I was telling him that I would go back to Switzerland in four days, he said: "I will return, too. I will leave, too."

We see with these last excerpts that despite the recovery of their children, parents still experienced concerns after their return. When we visited their home during a social follow-up about one year after six-year old Marek's return to Benin, his mother told the social worker that Marek was so rowdy and active that she was worried about his health and was afraid that his disease would resume.

CONCLUSIVE PERSPECTIVES: A COMPLEX EMOTIONAL NETWORK

In this chapter, I mainly focused on the emotions of children, their families, NGO professionals, and myself. However, all those who work closely with these children during the preparation of their medical travel, their actual stay, or the long-term monitoring of their medical and social trajectory, undertake a complex work of care, dotted with diverse and varied emotions. We have seen that important emotional work was undertaken within the work of giving care, by all actors toward each other during the trajectory of these children: by NGO professionals in Benin toward the families, by parents toward their children and by children toward their parents, by children among themselves, by medical, nursing and educational staff toward the children, and by myself toward the children. Each of these agents in the children's trajectory managed their own emotions at the same time as the emotions of others, recalling Strauss's understanding of the concept of a disease's trajectory as referring to the work deployed to follow the course of the disease, as well as the repercussion that this work and its organization have on all those involved in it (Strauss, 1992: 111).

According to Sakoyan (2010) in the context of the medical travel of children within the Comoros archipelago, inequalities can be found both in relation to accessing medical care (which refers more to the concept of *cure*), and in relation to social recognition and psychosocial *care*, such as benefiting from the presence of significant others, or having the possibility to communicate in one's own language. In the context of my study, it seems that, through their interactions with other children as well as with all the people who participated in their trajectory, some children have succeeded in reducing inequalities in terms of *care* as a mirror reaction to the filling of the need for access to the technical *cure* of their disease which the program addresses. However, as I indicated at the beginning of this chapter, it should not be overlooked that the very existence of this program is marked by profound inequalities in access to care which inevitably shape the children's experiences and which they are not able to respond to.

As such, it is important to notice that, although some of the emotions discussed in this chapter related to the diagnosis of a heart defect in children, and were, therefore, not directly related to their medical travel as such, many other emotions and situations of care arose specifically from this unequal access to care and to the specific context generated by it, and would probably not have occurred if the children were operated on in their own country. This is the case of all the emotions generated by the separation of children from their families, and the parental substitution work that resulted from it, as well as the emotions and additional work created by cultural differences and language barriers.

From a perspective of care ethics, this chapter reminds us that both autonomy and vulnerability concern all those who participate in the medical journey of children (Tronto, 1993). Zielinski (2010:636), relying on Tronto's work, recalls that the more care practices become visible, institutionalized, and recognized in society, the more attention to the needs of others will be favored, working as a virtuous circle in which the social recognition of care plays an educative part. This chapter thus contributes to the visibility of the care work and emotions of people, both adults and children, in the context of medical travels, with the hope that medical institutions and NGOs will consider the fact that care work and emotions contribute to the running of medical travel programs as much as protocols and technology do.

Finally, this chapter provides insight into different ways of considering childhood in general and childhood on the move (Vindrola-Padros & Brages, 2016). Indeed, it highlights traits other than the usual notions of vulnerability, dependence, and incapacity associated with childhood and children, by showing that they are also capable of taking care of themselves and others, adults and children alike, and that they develop many skills and strategies in order to adapt to their situation in a cultural and linguistic context different from their own. These skills include language skills, as they generally learn many French words and expressions adapted to each context in a few weeks, as well as cultural competences (Sobo, 2015) and educative skills, as they show a rapid understanding and adaptation to local manners and educative practices in their temporary home in Switzerland, and then readjust to the cultural and educative manners of their country when they return from their medical travel. As such, this contribution confirms that children are not passive objects of hospital and medical care, but that they can be actors in this setting (Mougel-Cojocaru, 2007). In the absence of their parents, children are thus capable of taking care of themselves, of their own medical trajectory, as well as that of other children.

REFERENCES

Ackerman, S. "Plastic Paradise: Transforming Bodies and Selves in Costa Rica's Cosmetic Surgery Tourism Industry." *Medical anthropology* 29, no. 4 (2010): 403–23.

Bochaton, A. "Recours Aux Soins Transfrontaliers Et Réseaux Informels: L'exemple Lao-Thaïlandais." In *Frontières Et Santé. Genèses Et Maillages Des Réseaux Transfrontaliers*, edited by F. Moullé and S. Duhamel, 145–65. Paris: L'Harmattan, 2010.

Bowlby, J. *Attachment and Loss: Separation*, Vol. 2, New York: Guilford Press, 1980.

Brannan, M. J. "Researching Emotions and the Emotions of Researching: The Strange Case of Alexithymia in Reflexive Research." *International Journal of Work Organisation and Emotion* 4, no. 3–4 (2011): 322–37.

Brousse, V., P. Imbert, P. Mbaye, F. Kieffer, M. Thiam, A. S. Ka, P. Gerardin, and D. Sidi. "Evaluation of Long-Term Outcome of Senegalese Children Sent Abroad for Cardiac Surgery." *Med Trop* 63, no. 4–5 (2003): 506–12.

Christensen, P., and A. Prout. "Working with Ethical Symmetry in Social Research with Children." *Childhood* 9, no. 4 (2002): 477–97.

Couturier, D. " Préface." In *Enfants Et Soins En Pédiatrie En Afrique De L'ouest*, edited by Y. Jaffré. Paris: Karthala, 2019.

Faist, T. "The Mobility Turn: A New Paradigm for the Social Sciences?" *Ethnic and racial studies* 36, no. 11 (2013): 1637–46.

Gallenga, G. "L'empathie Inversée Au Coeur De La Relation Ethnographique." *Journal des anthropologues* (2008): 114–115. http://journals.openedition.org/jda/319. DOI: 10.4000/jda.319.

Heinisch, P. P., L. Guarino, D. Hutter, M. Bartkevics, G. Erdoes, B. Eberle, C. Royo, et al. "Late Correction of Tetralogy of Fallot in Children." *Swiss Medical Weekly* 149, no. 3 (2019).

Hochschild, A. R. *The Managed Heart: Commercialisation of Human Feeling*. London: University of California Press, 1983.

Hunleth, J. *Children as Caregivers: The Global Fight against Tuberculosis and HIV in Zambia*. New Brunswick, NJ: Rutgers University Press, 2017.

Jaffré, Y. *Enfants Et Soins En Pédiatrie En Afrique De L'ouest*. Paris: Karthala, 2019.

Jaffré, Y., M. Diallo, V. Atcha, and F. Dicko. "Analyse Anthropologique Des Interactions Entre Soignants Et Enfants Dans Quelques Services De Pédiatrie D'afrique De L'ouest (Abidjan, Bamako, Conakry)." *Bulletin société de pathologie exotique* 102, no. 4 (2009): 238–46.

Johnson, G. A., and C. Vindrola-Padros. "« it's for the Best »: Child Movement in Search of Health in Njabini, Kenya." *Children's Geographies* 12, no. 2 (2014): 219–31.

Kangas, B. "Hope from Abroad in the International Medical Travel of Yemeni Patients." *Anthropology and medicine* 14, no. 3 (2007): 293–305.

Laurier, E., Lorimer, H., Brown, B., Jones, O., et al. "Driving and "Passengering": Notes on the Ordinary Organization of Car Travel." *Mobilities* 3 (2008): 1–23.

Lombart, B. . "Le *Care* En Pédiatrie." *Association de recherche en soins infirmiers* 122, no. 3 (2015): 76–76.

Lunt, N., D. Horsfall, and J. Hanefeld. *Handbook on Medical Tourism and Patient Mobility*. Cheltenham: Edward Elgar Publishing, 2015.

Marsters, E. . "« feel the Pain, Get on the Plane »: Cook Islanders' Experiences of Seeking Health across a Transnational Field." In *« transnational Pacific Health through the Lens of Tuberculosis » Research Group*. Report of transnational health research in the Cook Islands and New Zealand 2010–2012: Department of Anthropology, The University of Auckland, 2012.

Massimo, L. M., T.-J. Wiley, and D. Caprino. "Health Emigration: A Challenge in Paediatric Oncology." *Journal of Child Health Care* 12, no. 2 (2008): 106–15.

Mougel, S. "Des Écrits Au Sujet De L'enfant Hospitalisé: L'ouverture Des Services Pédiatriques Aux Parents, Une Histoire Méconnue." In *Les Enfants Dans Les Livres*, edited by M.-C. Mietkiewicz, 221–33: ERES « Enfance et parentalité », 2013.

Mougel-Cojocaru, S. "Quand Les Enfants Veillent « seuls » Sur Leur Trajectoire Hospitalière." *Face à face* 10 (2007).

Pirinoli, C. "L'anthropoogie Palestinienne Entre Science Et Politique: L'impossible Neutralité Du Chercheur." *Anthropologie et sociétés* 28, no. 3 (2004): 165–85.

Roberts, E.-F., and N. Scheper Hugues. "Introduction: Medical Migrations." *Body and society* 17, no. 2/3 (2011): 1–30.

Sakoyan, J. "Un Souci « en Partage ». Migrations De Soins Et Espace Politique Entre L'archipel Des Comores Et La France." *Haute Ecole des études en sciences sociales*, Paris (2010).

Sobo, E. J. "Culture and Medical Travel." In *Handbook on Medical Tourism and Patient Mobility*, edited by N. Lunt, D. Horsfall and J. Hanefeld, 217–27. Cheltenham: Edward Elgar Publishing, 2015.

Spitz, R. A. "Hospitalism; an Inquiry into the Genesis of Psychiatric Conditions in Early Childhood." *Psychoanal Study Child* 1 (1945): 53–74.

Strauss, A. *La Trame De La Négociation. Sociologie Qualitative Et Interactionnisme*. Paris: L'Harmattan, 1992.

Tronto, J. C. *Moral Boundaries: A Political Argument for an Ethic of Care*. New York: Routledge, 1993.

Vaucher, C. "Les Émotions En Tant Qu'outils Épistémologiques Et Éthiques Dans Le Cadre D'une Ethnographie Itinérante." In *Enjeux Éthiques Dans L'enquête En Sciences Sociales*, edited by M. Roca i Escoda, C. Burton-Jeangros, P. Diaz and I. Rossi, 193–212. Genève: Sociograph, Université de Genève, 2020a.

———. "Le Care Entre Enfants: Vivre Ensemble Dans Un Contexte De Médecine Humanitaire." *Revue des sciences sociales* 63 (2020b).

Vindrola-Padros, C., and E. Brage. "Child Medical Travel in Argentina: Narratives of Family Separation and Moving Away from Home." In *Children's Health and Wellbeing in Urban Environments*, edited by C. Ergler, R. Kearns and K. Witten. London: Routledge, 2016.

Vindrola-Padros, C., and G. A. Johnson. "Children Seeking Health Care: International Perspectives on Children's Use of Mobility to Obtain Health Services." Chap. 4 In *Movement, Mobilities and Journeys*, edited by C. Ni Laoire, A. White and T. Skelton, 1–18. Singapore: Springer, 2015.

Vindrola-Padros, C., Pfister, A. E., and G. A. Johnson "The role of anthropology in improving services for children and families: an introduction." *Annals of anthropological practice* 39, no. 2 (2017): 89–95.

Vindrola-Padros, C. "Life and Death Journeys: Medical Travel, Cancer and Children in Argentina." PhD thesis, University of South Florida, 2011.

Vindrola-Padros, C., and L. M. Whiteford. "The Search for Medical Technologies Abroad: The Case of Medical Travel and Pediatric Oncology Treatment in Argentina." *Technology & Innovation* 14, no. 1 (2012): 25–38.

Zielinski, A. "L'éthique Du Care. Une Nouvelle Façon De Prendre Soin." *Etudes* 413, no. 12 (2010): 631–41.

Index

affect, 8, 15, 65, 92, 126, 155, 178, 186
affection, 6, 14, 95, 101–2, 104, 155, 158, 166
affective attachments, 6, 171
affective practice, 4
affective relationship, 146
attentiveness, 6, 63, 95, 100–101, 104–15

carers, 7, 48–50
caregivers, 1–3, 5, 8–9, 36–37, 39–42, 44–46, 48–50, 187, 192, 198
caregiving, 3, 5, 7, 25, 35, 37–39, 41–42, 44–50, 67, 88, 100, 115–17, 133, 137, 162, 171
care work, 2, 4–5, 7, 9, 14, 22–23, 25–26, 28–29, 30n2, 31, 36, 40–46, 48, 92–100, 104–9, 117, 126, 131, 146, 165–67, 171–73, 178–79, 187–88, 191–92, 195, 197
Castañeda, H., 7, 82, 88, 116, 122, 135, 136
Crooks, V., 1–2, 5, 8, 35, 37–39, 45, 47–50, 73, 83, 86–87, 89, 92, 97, 110

Dalstrom, M., 4, 6–7, 9, 51–52, 66, 69, 72, 74, 77, 81–82, 87–88, 92, 97, 99–100, 110
detachment, 6, 158, 168–70, 172

diaspora, 11, 14, 17–18, 21, 23, 25–27, 29–30nn1–2, 33

emotional labor, 3–4, 7, 103–4, 184–85
emotions, 1–5, 95, 103–4, 118, 123, 136, 146, 158, 170, 174, 177–79, 181, 183–86, 188–90, 193–94, 196–98

feelings, 1–2, 4, 6, 103, 105, 107–8, 118, 131, 133–34, 144, 160, 187–89, 192–93
Finland, 2, 6, 18, 115–30, 132–34, 136–37, 139
France, 2, 6, 13, 16, 18, 28, 30n1, 51–52, 54–56, 59, 61, 63, 65, 67, 89, 179, 191

Greco, C., 2, 6, 9, 51–53, 55–56, 60, 63, 66n1, 67

holiday, 42
humanitarian aid workers, 6, 155, 158, 167
humanitarian organizations, 156

immobility, 57, 136, 139
India, 2, 9, 83, 89, 91, 93, 98, 108, 110–12

201

infrastructures, 4, 51
Inhorn, M., 3, 9, 53, 67, 73, 84, 87, 154
intermediaries, 4, 6, 27, 92
intimacy, 6, 155–58, 161–70, 172–74
Italy, 2, 6, 9, 51–59, 63, 65, 66nn1–2, 67–68

Kangas, B., 1–3, 9, 18, 32, 52, 67, 73, 81, 87, 177–78

Laos, 2, 7, 11–30, 30n1, 31n3, 32–33, 136
Lunt, N., 1, 9, 73, 88, 92–93, 106, 111–12, 153, 177

Medical travel facilitators (MTF), 5, 6, 74, 77, 78, 81, 83–85
mobility, 1, 8–9, 14, 16, 31–33, 35–36, 42, 45–46, 50–57, 59, 61–68, 94, 111–12, 115, 119, 133, 136–37, 139, 198
Mol, Annemarie, 10, 52–53, 62, 64, 67, 72, 82, 88
mutuality, 7, 102, 107, 118, 133, 172–73

networks, 6–8, 12, 21, 25, 41–42, 44, 46, 48, 56, 87, 110, 116–18, 124–25, 127, 129, 131–35, 137–39, 150, 153, 183

Ormond, M., 7, 10, 74, 88, 92, 94, 97, 100, 112

pandemic, 8, 54, 65

"patient-consumer", 112
proximity, 3, 5–6, 53, 74, 133, 135, 139

reciprocity, 7, 14, 25–26, 28, 31n3, 172–73
Russia, 2, 6, 116–17, 119–34, 136–39

Salazar, N., 52, 66
Sobo, E., 73, 81, 89, 97, 100, 112, 178, 182, 194, 197
Speier, A., 2–3, 10, 53, 64, 68, 73, 76, 82–83, 89, 94, 113, 146, 153
stuck in motion, 7, 116, 122, 135–36
Switzerland, 2, 5, 177–80, 183–88, 191–97

travel brokers, 2, 141, 142, 145, 151–52
trust, 6–7, 25, 52, 58, 60–61, 63, 86, 95, 106, 117–18, 129, 131–35, 139

United States, 2, 5–6, 11–17, 19–25, 27–29, 30n1, 32, 35–38, 40, 43–44, 50, 52, 66, 69–77, 79–85, 88–89, 137–38, 142–43, 145, 160, 168
unpaid labor, 4
Urry, J., 133, 139

Vindrola-Padros, C., 1–3, 10, 51–53, 57, 66–68, 83, 89, 143, 146, 153, 177–78, 180, 191, 193, 197–98
virtual, 6, 115

Whittaker, A., 3, 10, 53, 66, 74, 86, 92–94, 112–13, 149–50, 154

About the Editor

Cecilia Vindrola-Padros is a medical anthropologist working in the Department of Targeted Intervention, UCL. One of her research interests is the exploration of (im)mobilities in healthcare. She has carried out research on medical travel and has now started to explore micro forms of movement involved in the delivery of care. She is the lead editor of *Healthcare in Motion: (Im)mobilities in Health Service Delivery and Access* (coedited with Johnson and Pfister, 2018) and *Immobility and Medicine: Exploring Stillness, Waiting and the In-Between* (coedited with Vindrola-Padros and Lee-Crossett, 2020) and published *Critical Ethnographic Perspectives on Medical Travel* (2019).

About the Contributors

Audrey Bochaton is an associate professor in geography at University Paris Nanterre. Her work focuses on transnational health mobilities including patient movements, the phenomenon of medical tourism, and flows associated with traditional medicines and biomedical treatments in Southeast Asia.

Valorie A. Crooks is a health geographer and professor in the Department of Geography at Simon Fraser University (Burnaby, Canada). She currently holds the Canada Research Chair in Health Service Geographies and a Scholar Award from the Michael Smith Foundation for Health Research. For the past decade, much of her research has qualitatively examined the ethical and equity issues associated with the transnational practice of medical tourism.

Matthew Dalstrom is a professor of nursing research at Saint Anthony College of Nursing where he teaches public health and mentors graduate nursing students in community-based research and qualitative methods. His research draws upon anthropological and public health perspectives to study how health policy and the social determinants of health influence health-seeking behaviors, access to care, and health outcomes. He also collaborates with health systems, local governmental organizations, and academic institutions on health promotion research and interventions.

Joyeeta G. Dastidar is a hospitalist (an inpatient physician), an assistant professor of medicine, and a clinical ethicist at New York Presbyterian-Columbia. In addition to practicing medicine, she also pursued dual study in Narrative Medicine and Bioethics while at Columbia University.

Cinzia Greco is a Wellcome Trust Fellow at the Centre for the History of Science, Technology and Medicine at the University of Manchester. She specializes in the study of cancer and has further research interests in medical innovation, inequalities in access to healthcare, and gender and health. She has obtained a PhD in Health and Social Sciences from the EHESS and between 2016 and 2018 she has been a Newton International Fellow of the British Academy. She is the recipient of the 2016 Barbara Rosenblum Dissertation Scholarship for the Study of Women and Cancer.

Driss Habti is postdoctoral researcher in Karelian Institute, University of Eastern Finland. His recent funded research project is Career Mobility of Russian Physicians in Finland: Trends, Patterns and Effects (2014–2017). His research interests include global highly skilled mobility, international migration and ethnic relations, career research, immigration, and cultural diversity. He published internationally on these research areas. He recently published a coedited book on highly skilled self-initiated expatriation from multidisciplinary perspectives (2019), and an edited special double issue on mobilities and border research titled Engaging the New Mobilities Paradigm in the Context of Finland (2019).

Sarah Hartmann has a master's degree in Human and Economic Geography from the University of Zurich, Switzerland, and is currently writing her PhD thesis at The Open University, England. Her research interests center mainly on transnational space, networks, mobilities, brokerage, health geography, care, and care work. Transnational healthcare, medical travel, and particularly the work of different sorts of medical travel facilitators, have formed her research focus over the past six years. Her PhD thesis explores practices of medical travel facilitation in the context of south–south mobilities between Oman and India and includes extensive ethnographic research in both places. Following her interest in conceptual thinking, her thesis also sets out in bringing actor-network theory/STS and ethics of care into a productive dialogue.

Laura Kemppainen works as postdoctoral researcher in the Centre of Excellence in Research on Ageing and Care in the University of Helsinki. She also acts as a principal investigator in project Crossing Borders for Health and Well-being (funded by Kone Foundation, 2017–2020). She defended her PhD in sociology in 2014. Her research interests are in migration and transnationalism, aging, health, and inequalities as well as on mixed methods research. Kemppainen has published in international journals such as the *Sociological Review, Social Science and Medicine, Scandinavian Journal* of *Public Health*, and *Scandinavian Journal of Caring Studies*. Her book on Russian youth studies was published in 2016.

Elizabeth Lanphier is an assistant professor in the Ethics Center at Cincinnati Children's Hospital and assistant professor of philosophy and pediatrics, respectively, at the University of Cincinnati. Elizabeth received her PhD in philosophy from Vanderbilt University and her MS in Narrative Medicine from Columbia University. She also completed a postdoctoral clinical ethics fellowship at Vanderbilt University Medical Center. Elizabeth specializes in collective and shared responsibility, clinical ethics, narrative methodology, and feminist ethics. Previously, Elizabeth spent ten years supporting global health and humanitarian aid programs, primarily in francophone Africa.

Inna Perheentupa is a senior researcher at the University of Turku, whose research interests include sociology of health, civic activism, and gender studies. Perheentupa's doctoral dissertation is an ethnographic study on feminist politics in contemporary, neoconservative Russia (2019). Her articles have been published in journals such as *European Journal of Women's Studies* and *International Feminist Journal of Politics*. She is one of the editors of 'Assembling Therapeutics: Cultures, Politics and Materiality', a volume published by Routledge in 2019. Currently she is working on her own book, based on her dissertation, which will be published by Bristol University Press in 2022.

John Pickering is a PhD candidate in the Department of Geography at Simon Fraser University (Burnaby, Canada). His dissertation research has focused on international retirement migration.

Larisa Shpakovskaya is a docent of Higher School of Economics, St Petersburg. She defended her PhD dissertation in sociology in 2001. She studies gender, family, education, and social policy in Russia. At the moment she is involved in a number of projects on child wellbeing and reforms of the child welfare system in Russia. She also works as an investigator in the project "The layer cake of neighborhoodness" (funded by Kone Foundation, 2018–2020). Shpakovskaya is an author of several articles on parenthood, education, social inequality, family, and gender in Russia.

Mai See Thao is the Director of Hmong Studies and assistant professor of anthropology at the University of Wisconsin-Oshkosh. She is a medical anthropologist whose work examines the body, historical trauma, and chronic care. She has research interests in long-term care, health disparities, and immigrant/refugee communities.

Carla Vaucher has been employed as a teaching assistant and has been carrying out a doctorate in the field of medical anthropology. Her doctoral thesis deals with the trajectory of children suffering from congenital heart disease as part of a humanitarian medicine program in ten countries of West and North Africa. Through an itinerant ethnography, she is interested in the experience of Beninese and Togolese children, eighteen and younger, particularly in the way they understand their biographical and therapeutic trajectory, the identity reconfigurations they experience, and the strategies they implement to adapt to their cure and care away from their cultural, social, medical, family, and linguistic context for several months.